Ward Rounds
for
Medical Students

I hear and I forget
I see and I remember
I do and I understand

Ward Rounds for Medical Students

Clinical Medicine

GERALD SANDLER M.D., F.R.C.P.
Barnsley District General Hospital

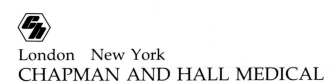

London   New York
CHAPMAN AND HALL MEDICAL

First published in 1990 by
Chapman and Hall Ltd
11 New Fetter Lane, London EC4P 4EE

© 1990 Dr G. Sandler

Typeset in 10/12 Palatino by
Best-set Typesetter Ltd.
Printed in Hong Kong

ISBN 0 412 30960 2

British Library Cataloguing in Publication Data

Sandler, Gerald, 1928–
    Ward rounds for medical students.
    1. Medicine. Diagnosis
    I. Title
    616.07'5

    ISBN 0–412–30960–2

To my sons, David, Jonathan, Mark and Peter,
all of whom know what it is like to be a student

Contents

Acknowledgements

I would first like to express my sincere gratitude to Alan Rogers of Knoll Ltd for his generous help with the artwork and also to Tracey Huddy of Stuart Pharmaceuticals Ltd for her help with some of the photographic illustrations.

I am very grateful to my friend and colleague, John Fry, for his helpful comments on reading the manuscript, and I am similarly indebted to my son, David, and my daughter-in-law, Clare, who have also read the manuscript and offered me many helpful suggestions for improvement.

Last but not least, I would like to thank my wife, Ella, who has spent many arduous hours with the word processor typing out the manuscript for me — 'Who can find a virtuous woman for her price is far above rubies . . . the heart of her husband doth safely trust in her' (Proverbs, 31, 10–11).

Preface

I often recall how much time I spent as a student in reading from cover to cover through, what seemed to me at the time, to be massive medical textbooks, with the admonition of my teachers — not to mention my student peers — ringing in my ears that I must read this book or that book if I hoped to have any chance of passing my final examinations. Apart from the inordinate amount of time and effort required to read, re-read and attempt to memorize the contents of these textbooks, I would often be left with no sense of clinical balance or perspective in what was common and therefore needed to be understood thoroughly, and which were the rarities that I would be unlikely to meet in future clinical practice but were nevertheless described, often in great detail, in the textbook. Another and even more significant problem was the undue reliance on medical technology that the books tended to inculcate in me, so that I was very wary of making any decision on diagnosis or recommending any treatment unless I had the results of the many tests deemed necessary by the authors of these textbooks. I now realize that not only did this approach debase the vital importance of the basic clinical skills of history-taking and examination in diagnosis and management, but the help provided by all these investigations was likely to be of very limited value anyway.

Regrettably, it has been my experience that similar teaching attitudes may still sometimes prevail. It is all too easy now to order a multiplicity of tests to the detriment of the use of the basic clinical skills in diagnosis and treatment. One of the prime objectives of this book is, therefore, to try to re-establish the value and importance of the skills of history-taking and examination in clinical medicine, and to do it in a way far more effective than the passive transfer of information from an author to a reader in the standard medical textbook, or from a lecturer to his audience in the medical school — by active, and inter-active, participation of the student in a ward round.

The other main objective of the book is to re-focus the student's attention on what the common medical problems really are in day-to-day clinical practice away from the teaching hospitals.

The book is based on ward rounds which I have taken with many generations of medical students through the years. It comprises twelve of the commonest medical problems which student and doctor are likely to encounter, and involves a dialogue between myself, the student and often the patient as well. In all the rounds the main emphasis is on the value and importance of the basic clinical skills, especially history-taking, since I am firmly convinced that it is a well-taken and perspicacious history that is most likely to give the diagnosis in the great majority of common medical problems. Appropriate investigations are also discussed in the various problems and their value as well as their limitations are pointed out. I have tried to highlight areas of inadequacy of clinical skills, knowledge, comprehension and balance so often repeated in the many medical students I have taught through the years.

It is my ardent hope that not only will this book help the student to pass his final examination in clinical medicine, but will also, and more importantly, prepare him properly to deal with the many common medical problems he will encounter in a life-time of clinical practice.

Gerald Sandler

1

Angina

Student

Mr M.N. is a 39-year-old salesman who was admitted as an emergency last night with chest pain. He was driving home from his office when he developed pain in the front of his chest with some aching in the left arm. He thought it was 'a touch of indigestion' since he has had a lot of heartburn over the last year and so he didn't bother to see his doctor. The pain got a lot worse during the night and his wife rang for an ambulance and he was admitted to hospital.

For the past few months he has had 'niggling' pains in his chest, sometimes on the left side, sometimes on the right side and occasionally in his back: the pains are often stabbing and just last for a few seconds at a time, but sometimes the pain can go on for several hours and there doesn't seem to be any relation to exertion. He admits that he is a worrier and said that his brother died last year of a heart attack at the age of 41; since then he said he was concerned about his own heart.

He has suffered with indigestion for about 3 years, mainly in the form of heartburn, and also complains of a lot of belching as well as a lot of 'rumbling' in his stomach. He has not had any problems with his bowels.

He has not had any other serious illnesses in the past but he did say that his blood pressure was found to be high a few years ago when he had an insurance examination but it hasn't been checked again since.

In the family history, I've already mentioned his brother who died young of a heart attack, and his mother, who is 63, has raised blood pressure. His father died of a stroke at the age of 67.

He has a very stressful job as a salesman and smokes at least 30 cigarettes a day. He is also quite fond of beer and drinks 2 or 3 pints most days and more at weekends. He is not on any drug treatment at present apart from what he has had since coming into hospital.

Consultant   That's quite a good history. What do you think of his chest pain?

Student   It sounds like it could be due to ischaemia.

Consultant   Do you mean angina or a myocardial infarction?

Student	I think that it is more like a myocardial infarction.
Consultant	How do you distinguish between a severe attack of angina and an infarction?
Student	The pain is more severe and lasts longer in an infarction.
Consultant	How long do you think an attack of angina lasts?
Student	It's usually about 10 or 15 minutes.
Consultant	In practice that's about right, but we usually say, purely on arbitrary grounds, that after 20 or 30 minutes we should start thinking of an infarction rather than an attack of angina. How long did Mr N.'s chest pain last?
Student	I'm sorry, I didn't ask him.
Consultant	Mr N., can you tell us how long your pain lasted when you came into hospital?
Patient	It was very bad for a few hours before I got into the Casualty Department and then they gave me an injection which relieved the pain very quickly.
Student	That would be in favour of a heart attack.
Consultant	Are there any other symptoms which could help you to distinguish between the two?
Student	The pain would be much more severe in a heart attack.
Consultant	Yes, and sometimes the pain is so bad that the patient feels that he is going to die.
Patient	I felt like that!
Consultant	Do you know what this feeling of impending doom is called?
Student	No, I don't think I've heard of this before.
Consultant	It's called 'angor animi' which means literally 'anguish of the soul'. Do you know any other features which would help you to distinguish between angina and a heart attack?
Student	He said he felt very sick.
Consultant	That's an important point. Vomiting is common in myocardial infarction but I can't say that I have ever come across it in an attack of angina. There is one other distinctive symptom which I think worth mentioning in angina and which was in fact part of the classical description of angina by William Heberden* in *The Medical Transactions of the College of Physicians* in 1768 — do you know what it is?
Student	No, I'm sorry.

* William Heberden, Senior (1710–1801) was a renowned English physician who practised medicine both in London and Cambridge. He was elected a Fellow of the Royal Society in 1748. As well as the classic description of angina, he also gave classic accounts of chicken-pox and night blindness.

Consultant	It's a feeling of suffocation in the patient's chest or throat — in fact that is what the word 'angina' means; it comes from the Greek. Do you know any other symptoms which might help in deciding whether a patient has had a myocardial infarction rather than an attack of angina?
Student	He was breathless.
Consultant	Why do you think that was?
Student	It's probably due to heart failure.
Consultant	That's right. Some degree of left heart failure is very common in myocardial infarction; it may be overt and cause breathlessness, or it may be detectable only on clinical examination or even only on a chest X-ray. Are there any other distinguishing features you want to mention?
Student	I can't think of any others.
Consultant	Dizziness is not uncommon due to impaired cerebral perfusion from a low cardiac output, and you can get palpitations due to cardiac arrhythmia which is frequent in a myocardial infarction; both of these symptoms are rare in an anginal attack. What did you make of Mr N.'s other chest pains over the past few months? Are they also due to myocardial ischaemia?
Student	I don't think so because they were not brought on by exertion.
Consultant	That may be of some diagnostic help but you must remember that anginal pain can also occur at rest as well as on exertion, e.g. during times of stress or excitement, or when a patient with stable angina becomes unstable and the attacks start to occur at rest. Is there anything else in the history which indicates that Mr N.'s chest pain is unlikely to be due to angina?
Student	It's in the wrong site for angina; his pain occurs on either side of his chest and not in the centre.
Consultant	That's an important point. Ischaemic cardiac pain is almost always felt across the chest, though occasionally it may be confined to the left side only. If the patient is able to localize the pain to one spot on the chest wall, usually on the left side and often just below the breast, it is not due to angina. What about the character and duration of this pain?
Student	Mr N. said that the pain was usually stabbing and would last only a few seconds.
Consultant	Angina is never stabbing and will always last longer than a few seconds; similarly, angina doesn't last for hours also — if it does sound ischaemic and lasts for hours then you must always think of a myocardial infarction. What do you think is the cause of Mr N.'s previous chest pain?
Student	I think it is 'musculoskeletal'.
Consultant	Not a very helpful term, though I know that it is used a great deal. What does it mean?
Student	I'm not really sure. I suppose it means that the pain is coming from either the muscles of the chest wall or from the spine.

Consultant	That is what it should mean but in the great majority of cases in which it is used there is really very little evidence of a specific lesion of either muscle or spine, and in my view, it is all too easy to delude yourself that you have made a meaningful diagnosis when all that you are in reality saying is that you don't really know the cause. I think that the best thing to do in this very common type of problem is to admit — at least to yourself if not to the patient — that you don't know the precise cause, but you can at least reassure the patient that you don't think the pain is due to coronary artery disease.
	Do you know any other distinctive features of this type of 'functional' chest pain?
Student	It's common in anxious patients.
Consultant	Yes, that's an important point and therefore you may well get other symptoms of anxiety like palpitations and breathing problems, especially inability to take a deep breath. Another useful clue is that the pain very rarely occurs during exertion but it may well develop *after* a stressful day when the patient is relaxing in the evening.
	Now you mentioned that Mr N. has had a lot of heartburn — do you think that this could be causing his pain?
Student	I suppose so.
Consultant	And what are the features of chest pain due to acid regurgitation?
Student	The pain is usually central but may radiate down the arms.
Consultant	You will find the radiation often mentioned in the books but in my experience that is very unusual too. What other distinctive features help to indicate oesophageal pain?
Student	It may be precipitated by bending and also by lying down.
Consultant	Good. Can oesophageal pain ever lead to angina?
Student	I don't think so.
Consultant	The relationship between oesophageal regurgitation and angina is complex. Firstly, the pain of acid reflux may be confused with angina; secondly, the regurgitation may trigger off an anginal attack and this attack may even be accompanied by ECG changes of ischaemia. Some cardiologists think it may be the cause of Syndrome X. What is Syndrome X?
Student	I've never heard of Syndrome X.
Consultant	There are three features to look for — typical anginal pain, ischaemic changes in the exercise ECG, and a normal coronary arteriogram: the cause remains a puzzle — it may be due to small vessel disease not seen in the arteriogram, a metabolic myocardial disorder or oesophageal dysfunction as I mentioned earlier.
	However, we do not think that Mr N. has heartburn currently so can I ask you whether there is anything else in Mr N.'s history which might suggest that he is a candidate for a heart attack?
Student	He is a smoker and he has a positive family history.

Consultant	The death of his brother was premature and this is therefore relevant. His father's death at 67 due to a stroke is not relevant since it is only premature vascular catastrophes in parents or siblings which constitute a coronary hazard. The smoking is a much more important risk factor, not least because of its reversibility. Are there any other coronary risk factors?
Student	High blood pressure in the past.
Consultant	Smoking and high blood pressure are two of the three most important coronary risk factors — what is the third?
Student	A high serum cholesterol.
Consultant	Good. Now if you wanted to distinguish yourself in your finals you might perhaps refine your answer on the cholesterol.
Student	I'm not sure what you're getting at.
Consultant	Is it the total cholesterol level which is the most significant?
Student	I think so.
Consultant	No, it is the level of the LDL-cholesterol which is the more important because it is this component which is atherogenic. The other main fraction of the cholesterol is the HDL-cholesterol which helps in the removal of cholesterol from the arterial walls. Therefore, the ideal blood levels to have if you want to avoid coronary disease are a low LDL-cholesterol and a high HDL-cholesterol content. Now, there is one other possible coronary risk factor in Mr N. — the stressful life style. Do you think that this is important?
Student	I think so because stress can cause myocardial infarction.
Consultant	I'll accept that but it does need a little modification. There is really no convincing evidence that long-standing stress can cause coronary disease but acute stress can trigger off a heart attack in a patient who already has coronary artery disease. Now I think we have probably got all we can from the history and it might be helpful to summarize our conclusions:

HISTORY

- the acute chest pain for which he was admitted is likely to be due to a heart attack
- he has several important coronary risk factors:
    cigarette smoking
    positive family history
    hypertension
- he has other chest pain which is likely to be related to anxiety
- he also suffers with heartburn probably caused by acid regurgitation

Consultant	Now I would like you to tell us your examination findings.
Student	Mr N. is lying comfortably in bed and he is not breathless. There is no anaemia, there are no enlarged glands in the neck and he is not jaundiced. The thyroid gland is not enlarged and the neck veins are not engorged. The pulse was about 80 per minute and regular, the blood pressure was 170/100, heart sounds 1 and 2 were present and there were no murmurs. The lungs were clear and the abdomen was normal. The nervous system was grossly normal.
Consultant	Are you happy with that presentation of your findings?
Student	I'm not sure what you mean.
Consultant	What have you learned from your examination?
Student	Well, nothing really — everything seemed normal.
Consultant	What you have presented appears to me to be a routine examination which seems to have little relevance to Mr N.'s actual clinical problem. Would you agree?
Student	That's how we are taught to present the examination findings.
Consultant	Yes I'm sure it is but don't you think that it would be a lot more helpful to present the findings in a problem-orientated way? The history shows that Mr N. probably had a myocardial infarction, and he shows certain risk factors which predispose him to the development of arterial disease. Wouldn't it be better to direct the examination and the presentation of the findings to establishing whether there is any evidence of atherosclerosis, to showing if there are signs of a heart attack and finally whether there are any complications of that heart attack? (Figure 1.2). So first of all what signs would you look for to indicate arteriosclerosis?
Student	You would check the peripheral pulses but I'm afraid I forgot to feel for them.
Consultant	Would you like to check them now?
	The student checks Mr N.'s femoral pulses and then the foot pulses.
Student	I can feel his posterior tibial pulses but not the dorsalis pedis pulses on either side.
Consultant	In the light of that finding is there any question you should ask Mr N.?
Student	Whether he has intermittent claudication.
Consultant	And does he?
Student	I'm sorry, I forgot to ask him. Mr N., do you get pains in your legs when you walk?
Patient	Yes, I have noticed an aching in the back of my legs when I walk uphill. I thought it was due to a bit of arthritis.
Consultant	That's a common misinterpretation by patients of claudication pain. What other signs of arteriosclerosis would you look for?

Student	I tried to examine his fundi but his pupils were too small.
Consultant	The fundi are very important when you are looking for atheroma since they are the only part of the body where you can actually see the arteries. If the pupils are too small to allow an adequate view then it is advisable to dilate the pupils but if you do this always make sure that there is no history of glaucoma.
	We will ask sister if she would be kind enough to dilate Mr N.'s pupils for us with some tropicamide drops and we will look at his fundi in a few minutes.
	Can we check any other arteries for arteriosclerosis?
Student	There is the radial artery but I find it difficult often to decide whether it is thickened.
Consultant	That will come with experience. There is another artery in the upper limb which may show arteriosclerosis — which one is this?
Student	Do you mean the brachial artery?
Consultant	I do. In well-established arteriosclerosis, especially in elderly people, you may see a very dilated and tortuous brachial artery in the arm — it is called a locomotor brachial artery.
	The other arteries which are affected by arteriosclerosis are the carotid arteries in the neck and the abdominal aorta, and you might be able to detect this by hearing a systolic murmur over these arteries — it is always worth listening for.
	Can the patient's eyes help us in diagnosing arterial disease? Now, I want you to look closely at Mr N.'s eyes and tell me what you can see (Figure 1.1).
Student	He has an arcus senilis.
Consultant	What is the significance?
Student	It suggests arteriosclerosis.
Consultant	In Mr N.'s case it also suggests premature arteriosclerosis because he is only 39 years old. It is of course a frequent finding in elderly patients who are likely to be arteriosclerotic anyway and is therefore of little diagnostic significance. What are those faint yellow patches on the inside of his upper eyelid?
Student	Xanthelasma.
Consultant	And what does that indicate?
Student	I think they are cholesterol deposits.
Consultant	That's right. This also indicates that he may have hypercholesterolaemia, which as we mentioned earlier is another of the major risk factors for atherosclerosis.
	I think we can see his fundi now — the pupils are well dilated.

The student looks at the fundi and states that the arteries look narrow and he can also see some arterio-venous nipping.

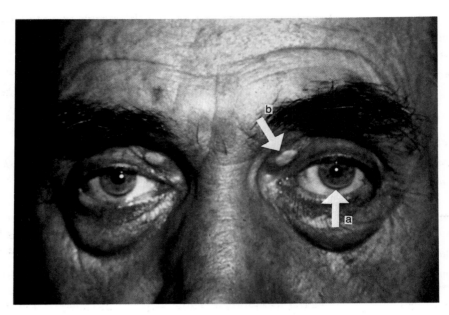

Figure 1.1 (a) Arcus senilis (arrowed) and (b) xanthelasma (arrowed) in a patient with hypercholesterolaemia.

Consultant	What do these changes indicate?
Student	That Mr N. has arteriosclerosis.
Consultant	Can we now turn to his blood pressure. You found this increased to 170/100. Do you think Mr N. has long-standing hypertension?
Student	He said it had been found previously at an insurance examination.
Consultant	That's true, but that may have been due to anxiety at the time — it has not been checked since. Do you think that clinical examination can tell you how long hypertension has been present?
Student	If arteriosclerosis is present this could be caused by long-standing hypertension.
Consultant	Good. Any other signs?
Student	I can't think of any.
Consultant	Would the apex beat help to decide about long-standing hypertension?
Student	Oh yes, you might get a left ventricular apex.
Consultant	A sustained forceful apex beat due to left ventricular hypertrophy would be suggestive, also a loud aortic second sound indicates that hypertension has been present a long time.
	I'd like you now to go on with the cardiovascular findings and tell us about his heart; what I would be particularly interested in is whether

there are any signs of a myocardial infarction — perhaps you can tell me what signs you would be looking for?

Student   There may be an arrhythmia.

Consultant   Arrhythmias are common in myocardial infarction but you have said his pulse is normal. Incidentally, you said his pulse rate was 'about 80'. I think it is better to be accurate by timing the pulse. What about the blood pressure in a heart attack?

Student   It is usually low.

Consultant   This can be the case especially if the heart is badly damaged. Initially, however, the blood pressure can be high as a result of sympathetic over-activity. Any other cardiac signs of a heart attack?

Student   The heart sounds could be soft.

Consultant   That's an important sign; the term we actually use is 'muffled' — this indicates poor myocardial contractility. What did you think of Mr N.'s heart sounds?

Student   I thought they were very soft.

Consultant   I would agree. This would support the diagnosis of myocardial infarction. Any other signs?

Student   There may be a murmur.

Consultant   What type of murmur?

Student   A systolic murmur.

Consultant   Due to what?

Student   It could be the result of heart failure.

Consultant   Yes, that's possible — it's due to dilatation of the mitral valve ring and is usually a soft blowing apical mid-systolic murmur which may be heard also in the axilla. Do you know any other causes of systolic murmurs in myocardial infarction?

Student   You can get rupture of the papillary muscle which causes mitral regurgitation.

Consultant   Good. This may lead to catastrophic left ventricular failure due to mitral incompetence and is an indication for urgent cardiac surgery. You recognize it by the classical loud pan-systolic murmur maximal at the apex and conducted well out to the axilla. Do you know any other causes of systolic murmur in myocardial infarction?

Student   I can't think of any more.

Consultant   Rupture of the interventricular septum is uncommon but can occur in the first few days after an infarction: it produces a murmur like mitral incompetence but sited to the left of the sternum over the 3rd/4th spaces. The consequences are not usually as serious as a ruptured papillary muscle.

	Now, I'd like to leave murmurs and go back to other cardiac signs in infarction — can you think of any more?
Student	You can get a gallop rhythm.
Consultant	Yes that is very important and frequent — what is a gallop rhythm?
Student	It's when you hear an extra heart sound.
Consultant	And what does it usually signify?
Student	It's a sign of heart failure.
Consultant	Yes, that's right. There are two types of gallop rhythm: a third heart sound — lup-dup-dup — which indicates either left or right ventricular failure, and a fourth heart sound also known as an atrial gallop or a presystolic gallop — lup-lup-dup — which indicates left ventricular failure or left ventricular strain in the absence of actual heart failure. What are the other two important signs of left ventricular failure?
Student	You would hear crepitations at the lung bases.
Consultant	And the other sign?
Student	Is it tachycardia?
Consultant	No, tachycardia does occur but it is not what I had in mind. The third part of what I like to call the diagnostic triad in left ventricular failure is breathlessness. Fortunately, Mr N. doesn't have a gallop rhythm and his lung bases are quite clear. Are there any other complications that we should look for in Mr N.?
Student	One of the other complications which can occur is shock.
Consultant	Cardiogenic shock is an important and serious complication. It almost always indicates extensive myocardial damage. How would you diagnose it?
Student	The blood pressure would be below 80 mm of mercury.
Consultant	What are the other diagnostic signs of shock?
Student	The urinary output is reduced.
Consultant	The figure we use is below 25 ml/hour — this is of course on a catheter measurement. What other signs are there in shock?
Student	The patient is very ill.
Consultant	Yes, that is true; more specifically, the patient is cold, clammy and confused. Do you know the haemodynamic reasons for these clinical manifestations of cardiogenic shock?
Student	I would say that it is due to a low cardiac output from a poorly-functioning myocardium.
Consultant	That would certainly account for the low blood pressure, the reduced urinary output and the mental confusion. What about the coldness and clamminess?

Student	I don't know.
Consultant	It's due to excessive sympathetic activity leading to an increase in circulating adrenaline — which causes sweating or clamminess — and an increase in noradrenaline — which leads to vasoconstriction and coldness and pallor.
	Do you know any other complications of heart attacks?
Student	You can sometimes get heart block.
Consultant	Yes, that's the other important complication. Is it more frequent in anterior or inferior infarction?
Student	I'm not sure.
Consultant	If I told you in inferior infarction could you suggest why?
Student	Is it to do with the blood supply?
Consultant	That's right. Inferior infarction is due to blockage of which coronary artery?
Student	The right coronary artery.
Consultant	That's correct and it is this artery which supplies blood to the atrioventricular node in about 90% of individuals, which accounts for the high frequency of a-v block in inferior infarction.
	To complete the important complications of myocardial infarction we should just mention emboli. Would you like to make any comments on this?
Student	You may develop a venous thrombosis in the legs which can lead to a pulmonary embolus.
Consultant	That is possible but not what I had in mind. Is there any other form of embolus that the patient may get in a heart attack?
Student	You mean a systemic embolus.
Consultant	That's right. Where might it come from?
Student	It can come from a thrombus on the heart wall.
Consultant	An intramural thrombus is common over the infarcted heart muscle and this is the usual site of origin of the systemic embolus. There is one other possible intracardiac site for a systemic embolus — and also a pulmonary embolus. Do you know what I have in mind?
Student	No, I'm sorry.
Consultant	If I told you that the patient had developed an arrhythmia prior to the embolus.
Student	You mean atrial fibrillation.
Consultant	That's right. The origin of the embolus is therefore in . . .?
Student	The atria.
Consultant	The left atrium for the systemic embolus and the right atrium for the pulmonary embolus.

Where do the systemic emboli usually end up?

Student I think that the brain is a common site producing a stroke.

Consultant Yes, I would agree that this is the commonest site. The other common site is the leg, and I have seen a number of cases of gangrene as a result.

At this stage I think we could summarize the examination findings and the conclusions we have drawn from them:

EXAMINATION

- Mr N. has a premature arcus senilis which suggests premature atherosclerosis
- the xanthelasma suggests hypercholesterolaemia
- he has mild hypertension
- the heart sounds are muffled, indicating some degree of impaired left ventricular function
- there is no evidence of actual left ventricular failure
- he had no arrhythmia, no evidence of cardiogenic shock and no embolic manifestations

---

Consultant Now turning to the investigations, what tests would you like to carry out on Mr N.? Before you give me an answer, let me say that I do not believe in indiscriminate routine investigation, a practice which in my view is all too widespread. I believe that tests should only be carried out to answer a specific question that can't be answered by history and clinical examination alone.

Student I was going to start by asking for a full blood count and urea and electrolytes, because that is the way we have been taught — to do these tests as base-line tests in every patient.

Consultant A blood count is of no diagnostic help in myocardial infarction, and similarly the blood urea and electrolytes are likely to be unhelpful unless there is associated severe heart failure.

What about electrolytes?

Student The potassium may be of help because a low potassium encourages arrhythmias.

Consultant I agree, but the other electrolytes — which are always asked for routinely — are of no help in managing myocardial infarction. The urea and creatinine levels may be useful to assess renal function in the presence of heart failure, or if you suspect renal failure as a result of long-standing hypertension.

What other tests should we do in Mr N.?

Student I think that the next test should be an ECG.

Consultant I agree. What would you be looking for in the ECG?

Student Changes in the S–T segment and Q waves.

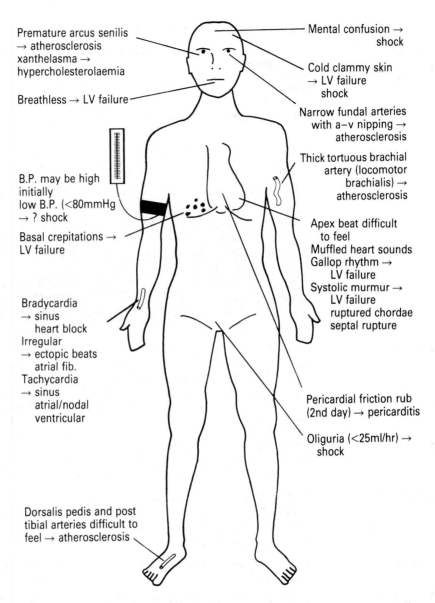

Premature arcus senilis
→ atherosclerosis
xanthelasma →
hypercholesterolaemia

Breathless → LV failure

B.P. may be high
initially
low B.P. (<80mmHg
→ ? shock

Basal crepitations →
LV failure

Bradycardia
→ sinus
   heart block
Irregular
→ ectopic beats
   atrial fib.
Tachycardia
→ sinus
   atrial/nodal
   ventricular

Dorsalis pedis and post
tibial arteries difficult to
feel → atherosclerosis

Mental confusion →
   shock

Cold clammy skin
→ LV failure
   shock

Narrow fundal arteries
with a–v nipping →
   atherosclerosis

Thick tortuous brachial
artery (locomotor
   brachialis) →
   atherosclerosis

Apex beat difficult
   to feel
Muffled heart sounds
Gallop rhythm →
   LV failure
Systolic murmur →
   LV failure
   ruptured chordae
   septal rupture

Pericardial friction rub
(2nd day) → pericarditis

Oliguria (<25ml/hr) →
   shock

Figure 1.2 Possible signs in myocardial infarction.

Consultant   That's right. There are three main changes to look for in the ECG in myocardial infarction — Q or QS waves which mean infarction with muscle <u>necrosis</u>, <u>S–T elevation convex upwards</u> which means myocardial injury and <u>T inversion indicating ischaemic</u> change only.
     Here is Mr N.'s ECG. What does it show? (Figure 1.3).

Student   The main change is S–T elevation in leads V1 to V4. There also seems to be some S–T depression in leads III and aVF.

Consultant	That's quite right. The other important finding is the QS wave in the anterior chest leads. Would you like to tell us what all this means?
Student	It means that he has had a myocardial infarction.
Consultant	Could you tell us where?
Student	The anterior surface of the heart.
Consultant	And which coronary artery is involved?
Student	It must be the left coronary artery.
Consultant	Could you be more specific and tell us which branch?
Student	I am afraid that I have forgotten my anatomy.
Consultant	In general I have not found anatomy very helpful in medical diagnosis except in two areas of practice — coronary artery disease and in neurological disease. In Mr N.'s case the artery involved is the anterior descending branch of the left coronary artery — it has produced what we call an antero-septal infarction. The QS wave indicates that the infarction is transmural, which means the whole thickness of the ventricular wall.
	What do you think is the significance of the S–T depression in leads III and aVF?
Student	It is due to reciprocal changes in the ECG.
Consultant	That has been the traditional explanation — that S–T depression opposite to the site of an infarction is simply a 'mirror image' of the S–T elevation at the site of the infarction: but there is now increasing evidence that these changes are due to multi-vessel disease: in Mr N.'s case this would mean involvement of his right coronary artery as well as his left.
	Are there any other tests that we need to do?
Student	Yes, I think we should measure the cardiac enzymes.
Consultant	That is the other important test. Which enzymes would you like to measure?
Student	The CPK, SGOT and the LDH.
Consultant	That's right. The level of creatine phosphokinase (CPK) is the earliest to rise, then the aspartate transferase (AST — formerly the SGOT) and lastly the lactate dehydrogenase (LDH). The cardiac part or isoenzyme of LDH, which is hydroxybutyrate dehydrogenase (HBD) is also measured. These enzymes are not specific for heart muscle and can increase in other conditions involving skeletal muscle injury, blood disorders and liver disease. You can improve the specificity of CPK by measuring its MB isoenzyme which comes almost exclusively from the heart muscle. Here are Mr N.'s results and you can see the considerable increase in all the enzymes over the three days during which we have made the measurements.

iu/L	CPK (24–195)	ALT (13–42)	LDH (240–525)	HBD (50–290)
Day 1	166	37	356	178
Day 2	1962	218	1394	715
Day 3	—	140	2124	896

Consultant	Are there any other tests we should do?
Student	I would like a chest X-ray.
Consultant	How would that help in Mr N.'s management?
Student	It might show cardiac enlargement.
Consultant	And what would be the relevance of that finding?
Student	I'm not sure.
Consultant	A chest X-ray is important in myocardial infarction for two reasons — it may show cardiomegaly, the significance of which is that it worsens the prognosis, and the other relevant finding is evidence of left ventricular failure. Do you know what the chest X-ray shows in left heart failure?
Student	You get pulmonary congestion.
Consultant	That's right. In the early stages, all you may see is congestion of the upper lobe veins: as the failure worsens the congestion spreads to the lung bases and in the most severe form of pulmonary oedema you will

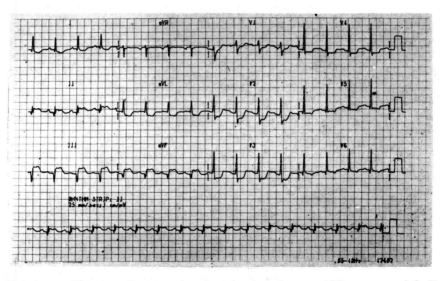

Figure 1.3 Electrocardiogram showing classical changes (QS waves and S–T elevation) of acute inferior infarction in leads III and aVF with so-called 'reciprocal' S–T depression in the anterior chest leads, V1–V5.

see the typical 'hilar flare' or 'butterfly wings'. This is an illustration of pulmonary oedema from another patient — fortunately, Mr N. had no evidence of heart failure in his chest X-ray (Figure 1.4).

Are there any other relevant tests?

Student   I think we should check his blood cholesterol level as he has xanthelasma.

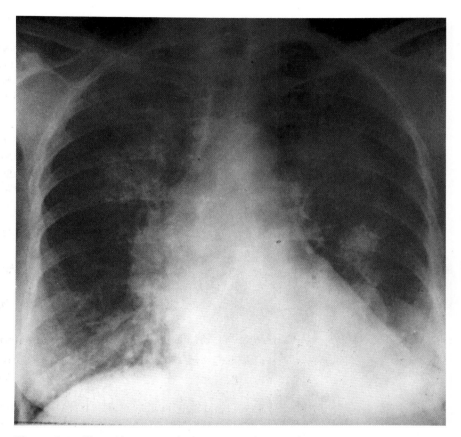

Figure 1.4 Chest X-ray in pulmonary oedema showing 'fluffiness' in the lungs in a 'butterfly wings' distribution.

Consultant   Yes, I agree but it would only be of long-term significance — it is of no value in acute management. In any case there is a controversy as to the validity of an acute-phase cholesterol measurement in diagnosing hypercholesterolaemia because the cholesterol level may be affected by various factors soon after admission like stress and recumbency. An estimation within 6 hours of admission is more accurate but it is probably best to wait for 4–8 weeks after the infarction to get the most reliable level.

Here are Mr N.'s cholesterol results:

		Normal range (mmol/L)
Total cholesterol	9.90	3.9–7.80
HDL-cholesterol	0.83	0.9–1.93
LDL-cholesterol	7.70	1.55–4.40
Triglyceride	3.22	0.55–1.90

You can see that he has hypercholesterolaemia as we suspected: more significantly he has an increased LDL-cholesterol which is the atherogenic component of the cholesterol, and he also has a reduction in his level of HDL-cholesterol, which is undesirable. All this bodes ill for his arteries.

Well, I don't think that there are any other essential tests for myocardial infarction — at least in a District Hospital like this. There are some sophisticated radio-isotope tests for picking out 'hot spots' in the myocardium due to necrosis in an infarction, and we did in fact do these tests here for a time but I found them of little practical use and they have been discontinued.

Now I think we should finish off our discussion on myocardial infarction by spending a little time on treatment. Would you like to give us your views on this?

Student	I think that the first thing to do is to control the pain with morphine or diamorphine.
Consultant	That's right. What would you do next when you have controlled the pain?
Student	That would depend on whether there were any complications.
Consultant	Before we come to the complications let me mention briefly that we are getting increasingly interested in trying to achieve maximum salvage of the damaged myocardium in the early stages of the infarction by active intervention with drugs like intravenous streptokinase and intravenous atenolol — we won't pursue this at present but you should be aware of this very important development.
	Let us go back now to the complications of infarction — which complications did you have in mind?
Student	The first is heart failure which I would treat with digoxin and diuretics.
Consultant	I'd agree with you about the diuretics but I would take issue with you on the digoxin, except perhaps in one important circumstance — which is . . . ?
Student	If atrial fibrillation develops.
Consultant	Good, but even then I think that there would be a better way of dealing with it if it occurs suddenly during a myocardial infarction.
Student	I'm not sure what other treatment you mean.

Consultant	Electrical cardioversion is what I have in mind if you can be sure that the atrial fibrillation is of recent origin. Why is that important?
Student	I don't know.
Consultant	Because of the risk of producing an embolus if the fibrillation has been long-standing. If you aren't sure how long the fibrillation has been present and the patient needs treatment because the ventricular rate is very fast then you can consider using digoxin but be careful because of the irritant effect of the drug on the heart muscle in an infarction; you might easily trigger off a more serious arrhythmia like ventricular tachycardia or even ventricular fibrillation. If you are thinking of using digoxin then there is one important blood test which you must always do first. Which?
Student	Do you mean the blood urea?
Consultant	No, that's not what I had in mind although there may well be a point in checking the blood urea especially if the patient is elderly — do you know why?
Student	Because digoxin is excreted through the kidneys and if renal function is poor in an elderly patient it would encourage digoxin toxicity.
Consultant	That's correct. But the other test I had in mind was measurement of the serum potassium level and I'm sure you now know why.
Student	Because a low serum K^+ encourages the development of arrhythmias.
Consultant	Right. What are the other complications that we have to think about in myocardial infarction?
Student	We've already mentioned arrhythmias.
Consultant	Arrhythmias are frequent and can be very important. It is helpful to separate them into brady-arrhythmias and tachy-arrhythmias. Could you give me some examples?
Student	You can get atrial tachycardia and ventricular tachycardia as examples of tachy-arrhythmias, and heart block as a brady-arrhythmia.
Consultant	Those are quite good examples. In fact, the commonest arrhythmia, which I would say occurs in at least 90% of patients in the early stages of infarction, is ventricular ectopic beats. I don't want to spend a lot of time on the management of ventricular ectopic beats as it still remains somewhat controversial. However, there is one type of ventricular beat which should always be suppressed and that is . . .?
Student	I'm sorry I don't know.
Consultant	The so-called R–on–T ectopic beats when the R wave of the ectopic beat coincides with the T wave of the preceding normal beat. Do you know why it is necessary to suppress them?
Student	I don't think I have ever seen any so I don't know.
Consultant	The reason they are potentially dangerous is that they may precipitate

ventricular tachycardia, or even worse, ventricular fibrillation — here is an ECG from another patient showing that occurring (Figure 1.5). Do you know what drugs we use to suppress these ectopic beats?

Student I think the drug of choice is lignocaine.

Consultant That is correct. There are of course a variety of other anti-arrhythmic drugs we use in the Coronary Care Unit including disopyramide, beta-blockers, flecainide and, the most useful of all for resistant arrhythmias — supraventricular and ventricular — is amiodarone. We could go on a lot longer discussing the treatment of arrhythmias after myocardial infarction but I think we should perhaps say a few words about another serious complication that we just touched on earlier — cardiogenic shock — because it seems to carry such a high mortality whatever treatment you use, but we have had some success with some patients. Have you any ideas on treatment?

Student You could use dopamine. — *improve renal blood flow + dobutamine - combination*

Consultant Dopamine is an inotropic drug and stimulates myocardial contraction. The other drug we use is dobutamine which doesn't accelerate the heart as much as dopamine.

Student Would you also use diuretics if the patient has left ventricular failure?

Consultant If that is necessary it is essential to monitor the left atrial pressure to assess accurately the response of the left ventricle to the various drugs because the patient is in such a critical condition. Do you know how we do this?

Student With a Swan–Ganz* catheter.

Consultant That's right. There is other treatment available which can help in cardiogenic shock, like angiotensin-converting enzyme inhibitors and intravenous nitrate but I don't want to pursue this further at present as it is perhaps a bit too specialized for your purposes.

I think we'll finish the management of myocardial infarction by considering briefly the long-term treatment. Do you have any views on this?

Student He should stop smoking.

Consultant That is vital, as it will reduce his chances of getting another heart attack.

Is there any other treatment which would also achieve this?

Student Yes, beta-blockers.

Consultant That's right. Unless there is any definite contraindication then I think that all patients should go on long-term beta-blockade after a heart attack; it will reduce the chance of a second heart attack by 20 to 25%. Do you have any other suggestions for Mr N.'s long-term management?

---

* H.J.C. Swan is a contemporary American cardiologist who works at the Cedars of Lebanon Hospital in Los Angeles; W. Ganz is a contemporary American engineer who works with Dr Swan at the same hospital.

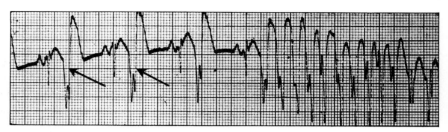

Figure 1.5 Electrocardiogram showing R–on–T ventricular beats (arrowed) triggering-off ventricular fibrillation.

Student	He should try to exercise regularly.
Consultant	That's a good suggestion though to be frank there is no convincing evidence that it will reduce the risk of another heart attack. A formal coronary rehabilitation programme is also very helpful after a heart attack, not only to improve physical fitness, but, more importantly, because it boosts confidence and morale which is often shattered when a patient has a heart attack. Now, I wonder if I can ask you about Mr N.'s hypercholesterolaemia. Do you think that he requires any treatment for this?
Student	Yes, I think that it would be advisable to give him a cholesterol-lowering agent.
Consultant	I would agree with you on this, but I think this not just because the cholesterol is raised but because he is only 39 years old. There is less indication to reduce high cholesterol in an older patient because the damage to the arteries has already taken place and it is unlikely that reduction of the cholesterol will provide any significant clinical benefit. What treatment would you use to lower the cholesterol?
Student	First of all he should have a low-cholesterol diet and if that didn't work he could try a drug like clofibrate.
Consultant	I would agree about the diet but we don't use clofibrate now because of its long-term hazards including an increase in mortality attributed mainly to an increased incidence of carcinoma. If drug treatment is required we would use a drug like bezafibrate (Bezalip) or cholestyramine (Questran). Other drugs for hyperlipidaemia include nicotinic acid, probucol and fish-oil preparations (Maxepa), all of which may be of value in resistant patients and may be used in combination with drugs like cholestyramine and bezafibrate. Finally, what are your views on the place of surgery?
Student	I suppose if the patient is young then he ought to be investigated to see if he needs a bypass operation.
Consultant	The fundamental consideration when making a decision about surgery in coronary disease is knowing whether the patient has left main coron-

ary artery disease or multi-vessel disease, both of which carry a bad prognosis. The only certain way of finding this out is by coronary arteriography. This implies that all patients with clinical evidence of coronary disease should have a coronary arteriogram; obviously this is not possible due to lack of resources so we have to be selective in deciding which patients should be referred for this test. Your suggestion of referring young patients is a good one and on this basis Mr N. will be referred.

One other useful way of selecting suitable patients is by exercise electrocardiography — those that have definite ischaemic changes are referred for arteriography especially if the changes are in both anterior and posterior leads suggesting multi-vessel disease.

OUTCOME

Mr N. made an uneventful recovery from his myocardial infarction.

He subsequently went through an intensive coronary rehabilitation course for 6 weeks which he managed without difficulty.

He was referred for coronary arteriography in view of his age. This confirmed the obstruction of the anterior descending branch of the left coronary artery, which was responsible for the anteroseptal infarction, but also showed 75% occlusion in both the circumflex artery and the right coronary artery. Coronary bypass surgery was considered necessary and was carried out successfully 8 months later.

LEARNING POINTS

Differentiation between anginal pain and infarction pain

	Angina	*Infarction*
Severity	mild to severe	usually very severe
Precipitation	exertion	rest — often in bed
	anxiety	stress may trigger
	cold wind	
Site/radiation	same	same
Effect of trinitrin	relief	no relief
Duration	up to 30 min	>30 min
Accompanying	suffocation	angor animi
symptoms	belching	nausea/vomiting
		sweating
		breathlessness

Characteristics of 'functional' chest pain

- stabbing or continuous ache
- may last a few seconds or several hours
- usually left inframammary
- unrelated to exertion
- other anxiety symptoms
    hyperventilation
    palpitations
    sweating
    tremors.

Relationship between oesophageal pain and angina

- oesophagitis may precipitate true angina
- oesophageal pain may simulate angina
- oesophageal disorder may be cause of Syndrome X
- oesophagitis and angina may commonly co-exist.

Features of Syndrome X

- typical anginal pain
- ischaemic changes in exercise ECG
- normal coronary arteriogram.

Coronary risk factors

- Major
    smoking
    hypertension
    high blood cholesterol
- Other
    family history of premature cardiovascular disease

diabetes
obesity
contraceptive pill
'soft' water　-
raised blood uric acid level
? stress
? lack of physical activity.

ECG changes in myocardial infarction

- T inversion　　— myocardial ischaemia
- S–T elevation — myocardial injury
- QR wave　　　— intramural myocardial necrosis
- QS wave　　　— transmural myocardial necrosis.

Cardiac enzyme changes in myocardial infarction

Enzyme*	Starts	Peaks	Ends
CPK	4–6hr	12 hr	72 hr
AST	12 hr	1–2 days	5 days
LDH	12 hr	2–3 days	7 days

* CPK — creatine phosphokinase
  AST — aspartate aminotransferase (formerly glutamic oxalo-acetic transaminase)
  LDH — lactate dehydrogenase.

Troponin I, T

Chest X-ray changes in left ventricular failure

- upper lobe venous congestion
- basal congestion
- diffuse patchy shadowing
- 'hilar flare' ('butterfly wings').

Relevant investigations in myocardial infarction

- ECG
- cardiac enzyme levels
- chest X-ray
    cardiac enlargement
    pulmonary congestion (LVF)
- serum K level
    hypokalaemia → arrhythmias.

Features of cardiogenic shock

- low blood pressure — systolic < 80 mmHg
- mental confusion

- cold clammy skin
- tachycardia
- oliguria — less than 25 ml/hr.

Indications for coronary arteriography after myocardial infarction

- young patient — under 40 years old
- persistent post-infarction angina
- anterior and posterior ischaemic changes in the ECG (multi-vessel disease)
- positive post-infarct exercise test
    anterior ischaemia — may mean left main stem disease
    anterior and posterior changes — multi-vessel disease.

Complications of myocardial infarction

- arrhythmias
- left ventricular failure
- right ventricular failure — much less common
- cardiogenic shock
- heart block
- papillary muscle rupture → mitral regurgitation and LVF
- septal rupture → LVF
- emboli e.g. brain → stroke
                 leg → gangrene
- SUDDEN DEATH.

2

Breathlessness

Student

This is a patient who has been admitted because of increasing shortness of breath. Mr N.W. is a retired miner of 59 years of age who has suffered from bronchitis for many years, but over the last few months his breathing has got a lot worse so that he can now do very little. Also, he has noticed on one or two occasions recently, that he has awakened in the middle of the night very breathless and he thinks this is getting more frequent.

In the past history I've already mentioned that he has a lot of trouble with his chest and often gets attacks of bronchitis, especially in the winter; he puts this down to having worked as a miner for nearly 40 years and most of this time has been spent at the coal face. He told me that he had to take early retirement from his job because of his chest problems.

On systematic enquiry he admitted to having pain in his chest which comes on with walking, and he has noticed this for the last year or two but it has not troubled him much recently because his walking has been very much restricted by his breathing problems. Another complaint on direct enquiry was that he also used to get pain in the back of his legs on walking, especially uphill, but this also is not much of a problem now because of the very limited walking. He has occasional swelling of his ankles which he thinks is more persistent now than it used to be. Otherwise, there was nothing else of note on systematic enquiry.

In the family history, his father who was also a miner died of chest trouble when he was 62, and he has one younger brother who is aged 44 and is still working as a miner and also suffers with his chest.

Mr W. is a heavy smoker, 30–40 cigarettes a day, and finds it almost impossible to give them up though he has tried many times. He likes a pint of beer but finds that he can't get out now to the local working men's club because of the increasing breathlessness.

His present treatment consists of 'breathing' tablets which he takes three times a day and a Ventolin inhaler which he uses whenever his wheezing is bad, though he thinks this is getting less effective than it used to be. The other treatment he gets from his GP is antibiotics when his bronchitis flares up.

Consultant	That's a good comprehensive history that you have given and should provide most of the information we need to get a fairly accurate diagnosis. What are your initial thoughts on Mr W.'s problems?
Student	Can I tell you the examination findings first before we discuss the diagnosis because he has a lot of good signs which help with the diagnosis.
Consultant	I'm sure that is true, but as it is possible to diagnose most common medical problems on the basis of the history — and I think you will agree that Mr W. has a very common medical problem, at least in this part of the country — I would prefer you to offer us your diagnostic thoughts on the history that you have obtained so successfully from Mr W.
Student	Well, it sounds as if he has a chronic lung problem.
Consultant	What sort of problem?
Student	I think he has chronic bronchitis.
Consultant	I agree with this diagnosis, but we usually use a rather more comprehensive term to describe the condition.
Student	You mean chronic obstructive lung disease?
Consultant	That's right. As well as the chronic bronchitis, there is another important component of chronic obstructive lung disease, isn't there?
Student	Yes, you get emphysema with the chronic bronchitis.
Consultant	Right again! Can you tell us how you have made the diagnosis of chronic bronchitis?
Student	Because he has had recurrent attacks of bronchitis over many years.
Consultant	I agree that is quite a reasonable basis to make this diagnosis, but to be accurate, however, there is a more specific definition of chronic bronchitis isn't there?
Student	Oh, you mean a definition based on a daily productive cough?
Consultant	Yes, that's right; the actual definition specifies a daily productive cough for at least two months a year for at least two consecutive years. Does he fit this definition?
Student	I didn't ask him when he produces his sputum. Mr W., when do you cough up the phlegm — is it every day?
Patient	I usually cough up phlegm every morning, especially after I have had a fag.
Student	Does this occur every day or is it only when your chest is bad?
Patient	I should say that I bring up phlegm all the year round.
Consultant	Obviously then, Mr W. fits in with the definition of chronic bronchitis. What is his sputum like?
Student	He said it was thick.

Consultant	What about colour?
Student	I didn't specifically ask him about this, though I did ask whether he had coughed up blood at any time and he said he hadn't.
Consultant	Apart from blood in the sputum, do you think that the colour is of any importance?
Student	Yes, if it is green or yellow it indicates purulent infection.
Consultant	That's a very relevant observation in a patient with chronic obstructive lung disease; in the absence of infection the sputum is usually grey or white. You mentioned haemoptysis; what would be the significance of this in Mr W.?
Student	It would indicate the possibility of a bronchial neoplasm.
Consultant	Yes, that's a very important consideration in Mr W., especially as he has been such a heavy smoker for a long time. Do you think that Mr W. has emphysema as well as chronic bronchitis?
Student	I certainly found evidence of this on examination.
Consultant	Remember we are discussing the history now so your examination findings are irrelevant at this time. What I'm really asking is whether you can diagnose emphysema from the patient's history?
Student	Well, it's quite likely because chronic bronchitis is so often associated with emphysema, but I am not sure whether there are any specific symptoms of emphysema as opposed to chronic bronchitis.
Consultant	No, there are no special symptoms specific for emphysema, but if a patient with chronic lung disease is severely disabled by breathlessness this is highly suggestive of associated emphysema. Uncomplicated chronic bronchitis does not usually cause disabling dyspnoea except, perhaps, when acute exacerbations occur. How severely is Mr W. disabled by his breathlessness? Mr W., perhaps you can tell us how bad your breathing is — how does it limit your activities?
Patient	It has been very bad. I used to be able to go to the shops and the pub which are only a few hundred yards away from where I live, but now I find that I have to stop after every few yards to catch my breath. We have also had to bring my bed downstairs because I couldn't manage the stairs.
Consultant	That would make it very likely that Mr W. is handicapped by emphysema as well as bronchitis. We will no doubt hear more about this when you tell us your examination findings. Now, let's consider another important diagnosis you should always think of in a miner who develops a serious lung problem.
Student	He may have developed pneumoconiosis.

Consultant	That's right. Do you think that pneumoconiosis can produce the degree of disablement shown by Mr W.?
Student	I would think so because it can cause extensive fibrosis in the lungs.
Consultant	It can indeed progress to massive fibrosis in the lungs, but this occurs in only a relatively small proportion of patients with pneumoconiosis.

Most of the patients affected have so-called 'simple' pneumoconiosis, which is a diagnosis made on the basis of the X-ray changes in the lungs — Grade 1 is a few small rounded opacities; Grade 2 more numerous opacities with normal lung markings, while Grade 3 is very numerous opacities with loss of lung marking. It is only in Grade 3 that you get a significant incidence of massive fibrosis — about 30%.

We obviously need to keep this diagnosis in mind for Mr W.

Now, I would like to turn to another important aspect of Mr W.'s breathlessness. You said that he sometimes wakes up breathless in the middle of the night. What do you think this is due to?

Student	It sounds like paroxysmal nocturnal dyspnoea.
Consultant	It does indeed — what can cause that?
Student	It's usually due to left ventricular failure.
Consultant	I agree this is a common cause. Is there any other cause?
Student	I think you can get a severe attack of bronchial asthma in the middle of the night as well.
Consultant	Good — that's what I wanted you to say. The next question, as you may have anticipated, is how to distinguish between what we call 'cardiac asthma' due to left ventricular failure and bronchial asthma, and I want you to concentrate on symptoms not signs for the moment.
Student	First of all, there may be a long-standing history of asthma.
Consultant	That's a good starting point. In Mr W.'s case, I don't think that there is any previous asthma as such, but as he has a long history of recurrent bronchitis and, in view of the relationship between this condition and bronchospasm, it is quite likely that his nocturnal attacks could be due to this.

What sort of past history might you expect in a patient whose nocturnal attacks of dyspnoea are due to left ventricular failure? What I'm really asking is the possible causes of left ventricular failure.

Student	Angina is a likely cause and Mr W. does complain of chest pain.
Consultant	Rather than saying angina as a cause of left ventricular failure, it is better to specify ischaemic heart disease since previous myocardial infarction, with or without angina, is even more important as a cause of the left ventricular failure.

Apart from ischaemic heart disease, what are the two other main causes of left ventricular failure?

Student	I think high blood pressure is another important cause.

Consultant	I would think that hypertension is the commonest cause of left ventricular failure. Can you think of any others?
Student	What about cardiomyopathy?
Consultant	That's quite an impressive diagnostic term! What do you mean by that?
Student	I don't really know much about it but I think that you can sometimes get hypertrophy of the interventricular septum which is due to cardiomyopathy.
Consultant	All that 'cardiomyopathy' means is a pathological condition of the heart muscle. It is usually divided, however, into idiopathic cardiomyopathy of which there are three main types — hypertrophic obstructive, congestive and restrictive — and secondary cardiomyopathy where the cause is known, such as alcohol, amyloidosis, sarcoidosis etc. I don't want to get diverted into a more detailed discussion of cardiomyopathy at this point, and while I accept it is a cause of heart failure it is not the third common cause which I was looking for — in fact it is a rare condition. Let me ask you again — what is the other cause of left ventricular failure?
Student	Is it rheumatic heart disease?
Consultant	That's right. What particular type?
Student	Mitral stenosis.
Consultant	No, mitral stenosis does not cause left ventricular failure. I have noticed through the years that students always bring it up as a cause. Mitral stenosis does cause pulmonary congestion and therefore acute breathlessness, similar to left ventricular failure, but the pulmonary congestion is due not to failure of the left ventricle in mitral stenosis but to the mechanical obstruction at the mitral valve leading to back pressure in the lungs. There is of course a type of rheumatic mitral valve disease which does cause true left ventricular failure isn't there?
Student	It would occur with mitral incompetence.
Consultant	That's right. The added load on the left ventricle from the regurgitated blood in the left atrium can eventually lead to left ventricular failure. What other type of rheumatic valvular disease causes left ventricular failure?
Student	Aortic valve disease.
Consultant	Could you be a bit more specific?
Student	Either aortic stenosis or aortic incompetence.
Consultant	Yes, both conditions lead to extra strain on the left ventricle and can therefore end in left ventricular failure. Incidentally, don't forget that there are other causes of aortic valve disease apart from rheumatism, such as atherosclerosis, syphilis and congenital valvular stenosis.

For the sake of completeness, we should also mention some other less common causes of left ventricular failure like thyrotoxicosis, congenital heart disease, myocarditis and, it is claimed in the books, anaemia, but I have never come across this as a cause of heart failure.

Let's get back to the important differentiation between cardiac and bronchial asthma. We have dealt with the past history; are there any points in the current history which might help?

Student	In left ventricular failure the patient can sometimes cough up pink, frothy sputum.
Consultant	That's a point which is also mentioned in the books, but in my experience, it is very rare that a patient will complain of this or even admit to it on direct enquiry, so I do not believe it is a very helpful symptom in diagnosing left ventricular failure.

What about the sputum in asthma?

Student	It may be thick and purulent.
Consultant	It would be purulent if the asthma has been precipitated by an acute respiratory infection, which may often be the case. But certainly, the sputum is often thick and difficult to cough up in an attack of asthma. When I was a student we had a name for the thick, stringy sputum in asthma which would sometimes resemble a cast of the bronchial tubes — do you know what that name was?
Student	I have never heard of it.
Consultant	It used to be called Curschmann's* spirals. It's another sign which I have not come across in clinical practice.

What is Mr W.'s sputum like during his attacks of nocturnal dyspnoea?

Student	I'm sorry, I forgot to ask him.
Consultant	Would you like to ask him now?
Student	Mr W., what sort of phlegm do you cough up when you wake up in the night with an attack of breathlessness?
Patient	I don't usually bring up anything in the attack, but occasionally when I have coughed up a bit it's not like the thick stuff I bring up in the morning — it seems more watery.
Consultant	(To student) What do you make of that?
Student	It's more suggestive of left ventricular failure than asthma.
Consultant	I agree. Are there any other distinguishing features between the two conditions?
Student	Does the patient sometimes get out of bed and stand by the window in cardiac asthma?

* H. Curschmann (1846–1910) was a German physician who became Professor of Medicine at Leipzig.

Consultant	Yes, that does occur, while in bronchial asthma the patient either seems immobilized in bed or sometimes he or she may sit at the side of the bed and try to fix his shoulder girdle by holding onto the bedpost or some other fixed object which helps him to use the accessory muscles of respiration to enable him to breathe. Can you think of any other differentiating points?
Student	No, I'm sorry.
Consultant	The bronchial asthmatic will wheeze a lot more in the attack than the cardiac patient, though in a really severe attack of pulmonary oedema you can also get wheezing due to oedema of the bronchial mucosa as well as in the alveoli. Let's get back now to the two other symptoms you mentioned in Mr W.'s history — the pain in the legs on walking and the ankle swelling. What are your views on these?
Student	The pain in the legs suggests he has intermittent claudication.
Consultant	I agree. Where do you think the arterial blockage is?
Student	In the legs.
Consultant	Yes, that is obvious! What I meant was in which artery of the leg?
Student	Probably in the femoral artery.
Consultant	The superficial or the profunda branches of the femoral artery are the usual sites of blockage with claudicating calves. What if the pain is in the thigh or the buttocks — what does this tell you about the site of the blockage?
Student	It means that the blockage is higher up.
Consultant	You're doing well. Thigh pain suggests involvement of the iliac arteries and pain in the buttocks indicates the lower abdominal aorta — in this case the pain is likely to be bilateral. What is the other important message from Mr W.'s claudication when taken in conjunction with the angina?
Student	I'm not sure what you're getting at.
Consultant	Do you think there could be a common pathological cause for both conditions?
Student	Oh, I see what you mean. Both of the conditions are due to arteriosclerosis.
Consultant	That's right, it indicates that Mr W. has extensive atherosclerosis, or, as we sometimes say, he is a generalized arteriopath. What about the ankle swelling?
Student	It could be due to heart failure.
Consultant	What type of heart failure?
Student	It would be cor pulmonale in view of his chronic lung disease.
Consultant	It could well be. Any other possibility?

Student	It might be due to venous blockage in the legs, because as I already mentioned he suffers from varicose veins.
Consultant	Yes, that's another possibility — we'll return to that when you tell us about the examination. There is one other very important factor in the history which is undoubtedly having a serious adverse effect on both his lung condition and on the arteries and this is . . .?
Student	His smoking.
Consultant	That's right and I am sure that Mr W. appreciates this. At this point, I think we have got all we need from the history and so we can try to summarize our conclusions:

HISTORY

- Mr W. has symptoms of chronic obstructive lung disease
- the attacks of nocturnal dyspnoea are more likely to be due to left ventricular failure than to the lung disease
- his ankle swelling could be due to cor pulmonale
- he has evidence of extensive arteriosclerosis manifesting itself in angina as well as intermittent claudication
- his heavy smoking is an important adverse factor in relation to both the lung disease and the arterial disease, and we mustn't forget the possibility of bronchial neoplasia

Consultant	Now, I would like to hear your examination findings and I want you to keep in mind the diagnoses that we have made on the basis of the history; try to present the findings in relation to these diagnoses (Figure 2.1).
Student	Mr W. is propped up in bed and slightly breathless. He is also cyanosed.
Consultant	Do you think it is peripheral or central cyanosis?
Student	His lips are blue and his tongue is also blue, so I think he has central cyanosis.
Consultant	What is the cause?
Student	It's due to the chronic lung disease.
Consultant	How would you recognize peripheral cyanosis?
Student	His fingers and toes would be blue but not his tongue.
Consultant	The face can also be affected in peripheral cyanosis, particularly the nose and ears. You will remember that cyanosis is due to an increased circulation of reduced haemoglobin — what figure is usually quoted for the amount of reduced haemoglobin?
Student	I think that it's about 5 g/dl.

Consultant	That's right, which means that you cannot see cyanosis in an anaemic patient with a haemoglobin of less than 5 g/dl.
	What is the cause of peripheral cyanosis?
Student	I suppose it is due to peripheral vascular disease.
Consultant	This can be the cause, but the commonest condition leading to peripheral cyanosis that you are likely to see is right ventricular failure.
	In chronic obstructive lung disease a distinction is often made between the so-called 'pink puffer' and the 'blue bloater'. Which do you think Mr W. is and can you remind us briefly of the differentiating features?
Student	I would say that Mr W. is a 'blue bloater' because he is cyanosed.
	I think the main differentiating point is that the 'blue bloater' develops cor pulmonale and that's why he is blue, while the 'pink puffer' mainly has emphysema without failure.
Consultant	That's very good. The 'pink puffer' is always hyperventilating due to emphysema and remains well-oxygenated while the 'blue bloater' has inadequate ventilation and is more prone to cor pulmonale; when this occurs the prognosis is correspondingly more adverse. The main pathology in the 'blue bloater' is chronic bronchitis.
	Forgive me for interrupting the presentation of your findings — please go on.
Student	His pulse was 100 and regular, the blood pressure was 170/105 and I couldn't feel his apex beat because of his emphysematous chest. I had difficulty also hearing his heart sounds because of the added sounds in his lungs.
Consultant	Before we come to your cardiac findings, there are two other important general signs you should look for in a patient like Mr W. who has been a heavy smoker for so long and has a recent deterioration in his breathing — we mentioned this condition in our discussion on the history.
Student	Yes, of course, I'm sorry. He didn't have finger clubbing.
Consultant	And what would be the significance of this in Mr W.?
Student	It might indicate a bronchial neoplasm.
Consultant	That's right, though it wouldn't be specific because clubbing can occur also in chronic obstructive lung disease as a result of associated chronic suppurative infection, like bronchiectasis, or as a consequence of fibrosis.
	The other sign I referred to is more specific for bronchial neoplasm.
Student	Do you mean lymphadenopathy?
Consultant	That's right — either in the axillae or in the neck.
Student	I checked him for neck glands and there were none. I'm afraid I forgot to feel in his axillae.
Consultant	Try to remember next time.

	The other important observation to make in Mr W. is whether he has cor pulmonale — the history was suggestive of this.
Student	I was coming to his ankle swelling next. He does have some pitting oedema of his ankles, and I thought also that his neck veins were distended.
Consultant	I'm glad you linked these two signs. What is their significance?
Student	It means that Mr W. has evidence of right ventricular failure.
Consultant	That's right. Can I ask you what the third important sign of right ventricular failure would be?
Student	Congestion of the liver. I could feel Mr W.'s liver but not very well because he doesn't relax his abdomen well.
Consultant	Try always to mention the triad of distended neck veins, congested liver and pitting leg oedema together when considering whether right ventricular failure is present. You mentioned the difficulty in hearing the heart sounds — what would you be listening for if you could hear them?
Student	I would be looking for murmurs.
Consultant	What type of murmur?
Student	A systolic murmur due to mitral incompetence.
Consultant	And what would be the cause of that?
Student	Mitral valve disease, I suppose.
Consultant	That would be a coincidental finding since there is nothing in the history to suggest rheumatic heart disease. In Mr W.'s case a systolic murmur at the apex would be more likely to be due to dilatation of the mitral valve ring as a result of left ventricular failure. What other auscultatory signs would you be looking for in Mr W.'s heart?
Student	He might have a gallop rhythm.
Consultant	Good, a gallop rhythm is due to an additional heart sound and that would signify ...?
Student	Left ventricular failure.
Consultant	Or right ventricular failure — you can get a gallop rhythm in both. Do you know the difference between a gallop rhythm due to a third heart sound and that with a fourth heart sound, also called an atrial gallop?
Student	No, I'm sorry, this has always confused me.
Consultant	A third heart sound — lup-dup-dup — indicates heart failure, either left or right. An atrial gallop, which sounds like lup-lup-dup, also known as a presystolic gallop rhythm, can occur in left ventricular failure but also may indicate left ventricular strain without failure, such as might occur in severe hypertension. We mentioned the triad of features in right ventricular failure; there is

	a similar triad of important features in left ventricular failure — can you tell us what these are?
Student	Well, we have just referred to a gallop rhythm; what about crepitations in the lungs?
Consultant	Yes, that is another sign. What is the third sign?
Student	Is it tachycardia?
Consultant	Tachycardia does occur, but the sign I'm referring to is much more specific for left ventricular failure and more obvious — acute breathlessness, which is the third member of the diagnostic triad. Is the pulmonary second sound of any importance in Mr W.?
Student	I'm not sure, I found it difficult to hear also.
Consultant	You would expect an increase in the pulmonary second sound in Mr W. because he may well have pulmonary hypertension as a result of his chronic lung disease. Now, before we get on to talking about murmurs and gallops, you should really have mentioned another sign which you may be able to feel on palpation of the chest — a sign connected with the right ventricle.
Student	I'm sorry, I forgot to mention that I could not feel a parasternal lift.
Consultant	What does a left parasternal lift indicate?
Student	Right ventricular enlargement.
Consultant	Good, it is the result of the pulmonary hypertension which usually develops in chronic obstructive lung disease. Before we leave the cardiovascular system, I note that you found Mr W. to be hypertensive, 170/105. I do not think we need to pursue this further at present but it will need to be kept in mind when treatment is being considered. I think we should now turn our attention to your pulmonary findings.
Student	He has a barrel-shaped chest, expansion is poor, the percussion note is resonant and he has widespread rhonchi over both lungs.
Consultant	I'm glad that you are following the traditional order of presentation of chest findings — inspection, palpation, percussion and auscultation — but I'd like to take you up on a few points. I agree he has a barrel-shaped chest — what does that indicate?
Student	It shows that he has emphysema.
Consultant	That's right. You said his chest expansion was poor — how poor?
Student	Less than what I would expect in a normal chest.
Consultant	Don't you think it would be better to actually measure the expansion with a tape measure which would give you an objective assessment rather than a subjective impression? There is another relevant observation you should have made on palpation of his chest before going on to the percussion.

Student	Do you mean tactile vocal fremitus?
Consultant	I mean vocal fremitus — the word 'tactile' is superfluous. Did you check this?
Student	I'm sorry I forgot.
Consultant	Would you like to check it now? Perhaps at the same time you could also measure the chest expansion with the tape that sister has for you.

The student measures Mr W.'s chest expansion, which is only ¾ in, and then proceeds to palpate the vocal fremitus at the front and back of the chest.

Consultant	What are your findings?
Student	I have confirmed the poor chest expansion which is less than 1 in, and I couldn't feel any fremitus coming through in either lung posteriorly.
Consultant	This is consistent with emphysema. Now, you said that percussion was resonant; I'm not sure what you mean by this. Do you mean normally resonant or abnormally resonant, that is hyper-resonant?
Student	I mean abnormally resonant.
Consultant	It is sometimes difficult to decide about hyper-resonance — it will get easier with experience. In general, if you get a good resonant note at the lung bases in a patient with a history of chronic bronchitis it is likely to be abnormal due to associated emphysema. Another way of deciding about emphysema, which is often referred to in medical textbooks, is by getting reduced cardiac and liver dullness. In practice, reduced cardiac dullness is of little diagnostic help since very few doctors — or students — ever percuss the heart. Reduced liver dullness in the chest may be of more value providing you know your surface anatomy of the upper margin of the liver — do you know?
Student	I should know but I'm afraid I have forgotten.
Consultant	I think it is normally in the fourth right interspace. Let me try some percussion in Mr W.

When the consultant percusses the patient's lungs he gets a very resonant note especially at the lung bases posteriorly: he percusses over the heart and is unable to elicit any dullness at all: he percusses the right chest wall anteriorly and finds liver dullness displaced downwards to the seventh intercostal space.

Consultant	I think we will all agree that Mr W. shows convincing signs of emphysema so far. Now, you also mentioned scattered rhonchi, which you quite rightly attributed to bronchitis; did you hear any basal crepitations?
Student	I don't think that there were any — at least I couldn't hear them.

Consultant	I'd like you to listen again carefully especially at the lung bases — try to ignore the rhonchi and concentrate on whether you can hear any crepitations.

The student listens again to Mr W.'s lungs, and after what seems an inordinate length of time, states that he can in fact hear crepitations especially laterally at the lung bases.

Consultant	What do you think is the significance of the crepitations?
Student	It suggests pulmonary congestion.
Consultant	Yes, I agree. Mr W.'s crepitations can be called fine crepitations and this usually indicates pulmonary congestion. If the crepitations were coarse and scattered throughout the lungs, what would it indicate?
Student	I would then suspect a generalized lung infection, like bronchopneumonia.
Consultant	That's right — fortunately Mr W. does not have this. Before we leave the lung findings, we should mention two important causes of acute deterioration of breathing which we should always keep in mind in a patient with chronic obstructive lung disease — do you know what these are?
Student	I know that a spontaneous pneumothorax can make an asthmatic worse and I suppose it can occur also in chronic bronchitis.
Consultant	That is correct — it's usually due to rupture of an emphysematous bulla. What is the second cause of an increase in breathlessness in a patient like Mr W.?
Student	I'm not sure.
Consultant	A pleural effusion which is a common complication in cor pulmonale. Fortunately, Mr W. doesn't have any evidence of either of these two complications. Now, I think we have dealt adequately with the respiratory and cardiovascular systems. Are there any other findings you would like to tell us about?
Student	I don't think so — the main findings were in those two systems.
Consultant	What about his claudication?
Student	I'm sorry, I forgot to mention his peripheral pulses. I could feel both femoral arteries which I thought were normal, but I couldn't feel the dorsalis pedis or the posterior tibial artery in the right foot — I could feel them on the left.
Consultant	That confirms peripheral vascular disease in the right leg, and as we said earlier, the blockage is likely to be in the femoral artery. I notice you didn't mention the popliteal artery — that is often omitted because it's difficult to feel but I think it's worth trying. We can feel Mr W.'s

popliteal arteries but the right is distinctly weaker than the left; this also confirms the site of blockage being in the femoral artery.

Do you want to mention any other signs?

Student	I don't think so.
Consultant	What about the fundi?
Student	You mean for evidence of arteriosclerosis?
Consultant	No, I wasn't meaning just that, though it is obviously of significance. I was thinking of the optic discs in relation to his lung disease — do you know why?
Student	No, I'm sorry I don't.
Consultant	You can sometimes get papilloedema in patients with severe chronic obstructive lung disease — do you know when this might occur?
Student	I'm afraid not.
Consultant	It can occur if there is severe carbon dioxide retention with failure of the respiratory centre which you must always watch out for in patients with chronic lung disease of this type.

Would you like to have a good look into Mr W.'s fundi now with this in mind and let us know what you think — the pupils are reasonably well dilated at the moment?

The student examines the fundi and reports that he thinks the disc margins are blurred. When asked by the consultant about the retinal veins he said that they looked congested.

Consultant	The blurring of the disc margins and congested retinal veins suggest carbon dioxide retention associated with some respiratory failure. This will need to be checked subsequently with a measurement of his blood gases — we will no doubt come to this in a moment when we discuss the investigations.

What other signs should you look for if you suspect respiratory failure?

Student	You can get a tremor of the hands.
Consultant	It is usually described as a coarse, flapping tremor. Did you check for this in Mr W.?
Student	No, I'm sorry.
Consultant	(To patient) Mr W., could you hold your arms out for us like this?

The patient shows an obvious tremor of the outstretched hands, though it was not considered to be flapping.

Consultant	Do you know any other signs of respiratory failure?
Student	You can get a bounding pulse.

Consultant   That's right, and if you feel Mr W.'s pulse you will certainly notice an increased pulse pressure — it's due to the peripheral vasodilation which occurs as a result of carbon dioxide retention in respiratory failure.

It would appear therefore, that Mr W. does have all the signs of respiratory failure.

I think it would be appropriate now to summarize the results of your examination:

EXAMINATION

- Mr W. has evidence of bronchitis and emphysema
- he has mild cor pulmonale
- there is clinical evidence of respiratory failure as shown by tremor, bounding pulse and papilloedema
- there is mild hypertension with some basal pulmonary congestion due to left ventricular failure
- there is evidence of peripheral vascular disease with the site of obstruction likely to be in the right femoral artery

---

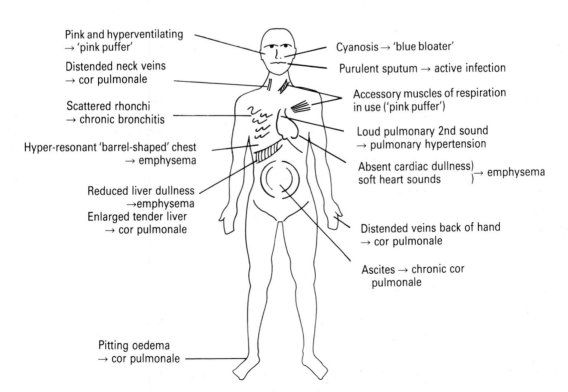

Pink and hyperventilating → 'pink puffer'

Distended neck veins → cor pulmonale

Scattered rhonchi → chronic bronchitis

Hyper-resonant 'barrel-shaped' chest → emphysema

Reduced liver dullness →emphysema
Enlarged tender liver → cor pulmonale

Pitting oedema → cor pulmonale

Cyanosis → 'blue bloater'

Purulent sputum → active infection

Accessory muscles of respiration in use ('pink puffer')

Loud pulmonary 2nd sound → pulmonary hypertension

Absent cardiac dullness) soft heart sounds) → emphysema

Distended veins back of hand → cor pulmonale

Ascites → chronic cor pulmonale

Figure 2.1   Possible signs in chronic obstructive airways disease.

Consultant	Now, can I ask you whether you think Mr W. needs any tests?
Student	I think I would start with a blood count and ESR.
Consultant	How do you think these would help in Mr W.'s management?
Student	He might have an increase in the white cell count.
Consultant	What would that indicate?
Student	It would suggest that he could have active infection in his lungs.
Consultant	Leucocytosis is a very non-specific test isn't it? Don't you think there is a much better way of deciding whether Mr W. has an acute lung infection — and it's something you can do yourself without the help of any other hospital department?
Student	You mean look at the sputum.
Consultant	That's exactly what I do mean — a very simple observation which is all too often neglected in favour of blood counts and laboratory investigation of the sputum. If the patient's sputum is green or yellow then he has a purulent infection in his lungs irrespective of what the white count shows. If, in addition, you weigh the sputum daily you will have a simple objective measure also of assessing his response to treatment. What other information would you be looking for in the blood count?
Student	It might show anaemia.
Consultant	I don't see why it should — in fact it's quite likely to show the reverse, isn't it?
Student	You mean polycythaemia.
Consultant	That's right — secondary polycythaemia as a result of chronic anoxaemia from his obstructive lung disease. Is this important?
Student	It could lead to thrombosis.
Consultant	That's right. Polycythaemia slows the circulation and therefore increases the chances of thrombosis. It is also important if the patient develops cor pulmonale because venesection would then be well worth considering as part of the treatment. You also asked for the ESR. What would you hope to learn from this?
Student	I was thinking that a raised ESR would help to diagnose infection in the lungs, but in view of what you said earlier about purulent sputum being the important thing, I suppose that the ESR is not necessary for the diagnosis.
Consultant	You have picked up the point well. Here is Mr W.'s blood count — perhaps you could comment on it for us?
Student	The haemoglobin and red cell count are high, indicating polycythaemia, and this fits in with the increased packed cell volume. The white cell count is also increased probably due to infection in the lungs.

		Normal range
Haemoglobin	18.9 g/dl	(12–16)
Red cell count	7.7×10^{12}/L	(4.2–5.9)
Packed cell volume	55 %	(45–50)
White cell count	13.7×10^{9}/L	(4–11)
ESR	1 mm/hr	(5–15)

	I'm a bit puzzled by the very low ESR — I would have expected it to be up also if there were acute infection in the lungs.
Consultant	The ESR is low because of the polycythaemia — the densely packed red cells are slow in settling and therefore you will get a low result. What other tests would you like?
Student	I think we should have a chest X-ray.
Consultant	Why do you want a chest X-ray?
Student	To confirm that he has chronic bronchitis and emphysema.
Consultant	Do you have any doubt about the diagnosis of chronic obstructive disease which we have made on clinical assessment?
Student	Not really, but I thought that a chest X-ray might show us the severity of the condition.
Consultant	The severity of his condition is probably best assessed on his symptoms, especially the degree of breathlessness. If you did want a more objective measurement of the disability there are other better tests which we will be coming to shortly.
	The main value of the chest X-ray in chronic obstructive lung disease would be to exclude other associated conditions like pneumoconiosis, which is very common in the Barnsley area, a pneumothorax which could greatly exacerbate the dyspnoea and also bronchial carcinoma, the incidence of which is increased in chronic bronchitis.
	Another useful point you could get from the chest X-ray is the heart size, which is important in assessing prognosis. There is one other change we would look for in Mr W.'s X-ray and that is evidence of left ventricular failure which we suspected from the history.
	Here is Mr W.'s chest X-ray (Figure 2.2). Would you like to tell us what you think of it?
Student	It confirms emphysema.
Consultant	Why do you say that?
Student	The lung fields are very dark.
Consultant	Right, there is increased translucency because of the overfilled lungs. Do you know any other radiological signs of emphysema?
Student	The diaphragm is low.

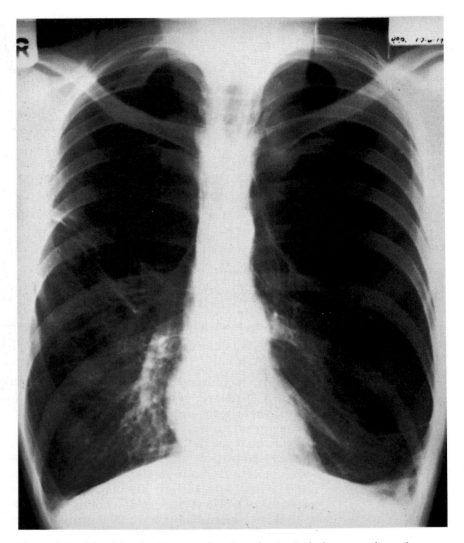

Figure 2.2 Mr W.'s chest X-ray showing the typical changes of emphysema with horizontal ribs, low flat diaphragm and over-translucent lung fields.

Consultant	Good; Mr W.'s X-ray shows it. Any other useful signs?
Student	I'm not sure.
Consultant	The ribs are more horizontal, the heart tends to be long and narrow and sometimes you may see some large bullae. Do you know what the X-ray is like in chronic bronchitis without emphysema?
Student	No, I don't think so.

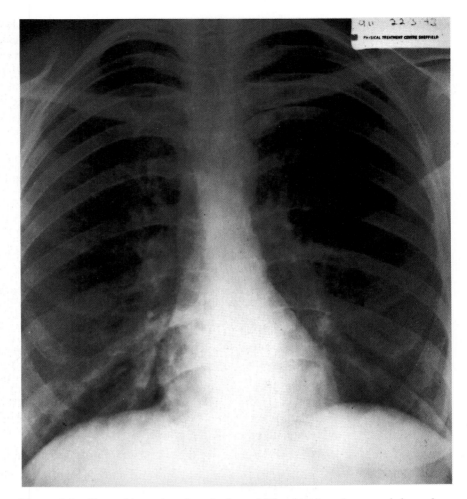

Figure 2.3 Chest X-ray in chronic bronchitis showing increased broncho-vascular markings at the lung bases.

Consultant	The main abnormality in chronic bronchitis is increase in the bronchial lung markings, especially at the lung bases (Figure 2.3). Fortunately, Mr W. doesn't have any of the complications in his X-ray that we mentioned earlier, and there is no evidence of pulmonary congestion due to left ventricular failure at the moment. Are there any other tests we should do?
Student	His sputum should be examined for pathogens.
Consultant	How would this help?
Student	It would tell us what kind of infection Mr W. has in the lungs.

Consultant	I'm glad you didn't say that it would tell us whether Mr W. has an infection in his lungs as we have already stressed that you decide this on the basis of the colour of the sputum, and not on whether you can show organisms in the sputum. In any case, in my experience, the sputum is often reported as negative for pathogens, even when there is no doubt about active infection from the appearance of green or yellow sputum. Another problem about relying on the sputum is that it often takes several days for the result to come through, and you cannot afford to delay treatment while you are waiting. Having said all that, the sputum may be of help if you come across a resistant infection which has not cleared with your initial antibiotic therapy. Now what about other tests for Mr W.?
Student	Do you think we should do an ECG?
Consultant	How would this help?
Student	It could show right ventricular hypertrophy.
Consultant	Yes, that is an important point because it would worsen the prognosis. Here is Mr W.'s ECG (Figure 2.4). Can we have your comments?
Student	There is a tall R wave in V1 as well as T inversion.
Consultant	Do you know what this means?
Student	I think it's due to right ventricular strain.
Consultant	This indicates pulmonary hypertension which is an adverse prognostic sign. You will notice also that he has a tall P wave which is due to right atrial hypertrophy, and is also a sign of pulmonary hypertension. Are there any more tests you would like?
Student	We should measure the blood urea and electrolytes.
Consultant	The blood urea might be useful since he does have cor pulmonale and this can depress renal function. The electrolytes are of no diagnostic help though the potassium level would be important if he was on diuretic treatment. Could we concentrate at this point on assessment of the degree of his respiratory disability — how can we do that?
Student	We could do pulmonary function tests.
Consultant	Could you tell us more specifically how this might help?
Student	It will confirm small airway obstruction from his chronic bronchitis — we could get this from the $FEV_{1.0}$, and it will also show how bad it is.
Consultant	Right. We could also decide whether the obstruction is reversible by repeating the $FEV_{1.0}$ after giving him a bronchodilator aerosol. The other important finding we could obtain from the test is whether there is also a restrictive defect from the associated emphysema in Mr W.'s case. Here is the result of Mr W.'s test which was done on a vitallograph:

		Predicted normal
$FEV_{1.0}$	1.1 L/sec	3.64
	1.15 L/sec	
	(after bronchodilator)	
FVC	2.5 L/sec	4.25
$FEV_{1.0}/FVC$	44%	70–75%

$FEV_{1.0}$ = forced expiratory volume at one second
FVC = forced vital capacity.

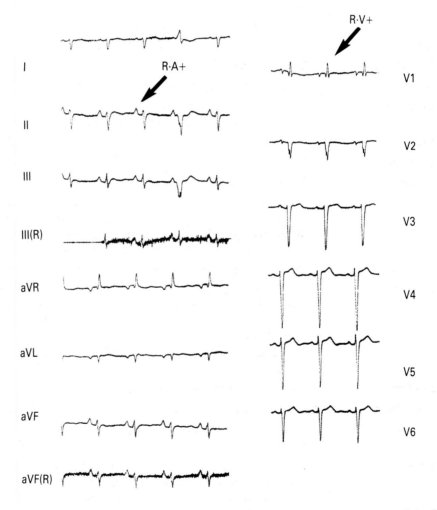

Figure 2.4 Electrocardiogram showing right atrial hypertrophy (arrowed) and right ventricular hypertrophy (arrowed) in a patient with severe chronic obstructive airways disease.

Consultant	You will see that the reduced $FEV_{1.0}$ confirms the small airway obstruction and furthermore there is no significant improvement with bronchodilatation — what does this mean?
Student	That the obstruction is not reversible.
Consultant	This suggests that it is not due to bronchospasm. You will also notice the reduced $FEV_{1.0}$/FVC ratio which is also typical of small airway obstruction. Finally, you will see the reduced vital capacity which is a restrictive type of defect and is due to the emphysema. These results confirm that Mr W. has severe chronic obstructive airway disease as we suspected from our clinical assessment. Now, there is one other very important test which gives us a good indication of the degree of respiratory failure associated with this type of chronic lung disease — do you know what it is?
Student	Measurement of the blood gases.
Consultant	That's right, especially the pCO_2 level. Here is Mr W.'s result.

		Normal range
pO_2	7.2 kPa	12–15
pCO_2	12.9 kPa	4.5–6
pH	7.3	7.35–7.45

You will see evidence of carbon dioxide retention, anoxaemia and acidosis, all of which indicates a severe degree of respiratory insufficiency. This is a very important test in the management of chronic obstructive lung disease since a progressive deterioration of these results with treatment is an urgent indication to consider positive-pressure ventilation.

Consultant	Well, I'm sorry but we will have to finish there because of lack of time. I would have liked to have discussed Mr W.'s management with you, particularly with reference to the four important aspects of treatment — control of infection, improvement of small airway obstruction, counteracting anoxaemia and treatment of cor pulmonale. Perhaps we can get round to it some other time.

OUTCOME

Mr W. was given a course of co-trimoxazole which reduced the daily weight of his sputum from 50–60 g to 15 g and changed the colour from pale green to grey. The coughing up of the sputum was helped by daily physiotherapy with deep breathing exercises and chest percussion.

Small airway obstruction, which was monitored daily with a peak-flow meter, improved from 95 L/min to 220 L/min with 4-hourly salbutamol by nebulizer; 28% oxygen was used freely through a mask, and the blood gases measured daily to assess response, which was satisfactory.

His cor pulmonale was treated with frusemide and the weight fell daily as the ankle oedema disappeared.

Mr W. was discharged from hospital after 10 days' treatment and was advised to continue maintenance treatment with:

- frusemide 40 mg/day
- beclomethasone inhalation 4 times daily
- salbutamol by inhaler when necessary
- domiciliary O_2 was to be arranged by the GP

LEARNING POINTS

Diagnostic triads in heart failure

Left ventricular failure
- dyspnoea
- gallop rhythm
- pulmonary crepitations.

Right ventricular failure
- distended neck veins
- congested liver
- pitting oedema of the legs.

Differentiation between a 'pink puffer' and a 'blue bloater'

	'Pink puffer'	*'Blue bloater'*
Breathing	noisy hyperventilation	quiet hypoventilation
Colour	pink	blue
Chest signs	emphysema — barrel-shape hyper-resonant poor air entry	bronchitis — rhonchi +
Cardiac signs	nil	cor pulmonale
pO_2	normal	low
pCO_2	normal	increased

Differentiation between 'cardiac' and bronchial asthma

	'Cardiac'	*Bronchial*
Past history	hypertension myocardial ischaemia valvular heart disease	asthma chronic bronchitis
Timing	any time	early morning
Sputum	pink and frothy	thick and gelatinous
Relief	getting up (window) diuretic	coughing up sputum bronchodilator
Lung signs	crepitations	rhonchi
Heart	gallop rhythm	nil significant

X-ray changes in chronic bronchitis and emphysema

	Chronic bronchitis	*Emphysema*
Translucency	normal	increased
Ribs	normal	horizontal
Diaphragm	normal shape and level	flattened and depressed
Lung markings	increased especially at the bases	attenuated
Pulmonary artery	prominent	normal
Bullae	none	sometimes
Fibrosis	sometimes	rare
Heart	may be enlarged due to pulmonary hypertension	long and narrow

Useful tests in chronic obstructive lung disease

- haemoglobin
    secondary polycythaemia
- packed cell volume
    confirms polycythaemia
- blood urea
    for renal assessment if cor pulmonale
- chest X-ray
    to distinguish bronchitis or emphysema
    for associated pneumoconiosis
    to pick up a pneumothorax
    to exclude bronchial carcinoma
- ECG
    for right ventricular hypertrophy ± strain
    for right atrial hypertrophy
- respiratory function
    indicates small airway obstruction and whether reversible with
        bronchodilator
    shows restrictive defect due to emphysema
- blood gases
    the pCO_2 level indicates degree of respiratory failure — important in
        assessing response to treatment.

Features of carbon dioxide retention in chronic obstructive airway disease

- throbbing headache
- tremor
- drowsiness
- fast bounding pulse
- fundi
    congested veins
    papilloedema.

Treatment of chronic obstructive airway disease

General measures
- *STOP SMOKING*
- reduce obesity
- treat depression
- regular medical supervision
    check sputum for infection
    check and treat cor pulmonale
    support and encourage
- home nursing service
- social worker's help

Specific treatment
- control infection
    antibiotics

- improve airway obstruction
  bronchodilator aerosol
  oral bronchodilators
  steroids
    aerosol
    oral
- improve anoxaemia
  oxygen
- treat cor pulmonale
  diuretics.

3

Hypertension

Student | Mr F.B. is a 64-year-old retired coal miner who presented with high blood pressure. He thinks it was first found 2 years ago and he has been treated with Adalat (nifedipine) since.

He has been unwell over the last few days with palpitations and dizziness, and over the last few weeks he has been unsteady on first getting up in the morning. Other symptoms include headaches with vomiting, and tiredness all the time.

There was a past history of a sudden onset of weakness on his left side 1 year ago; it lasted about a day and his GP told him it was a slight stroke. Also, there was a history of angina over the past year, for which he was admitted on one occasion when it was thought he might have had a heart attack. Other problems are chronic bronchitis, a 10-year history of indigestion and long-standing varicose veins for which he had an operation 3 years ago.

His current treatment consists of Adalat, Lasix (frusemide) and Tagamet (cimetidine) for his ulcer.

In the family history, his father and brother suffer with high blood pressure.

He smokes 20 to 30 cigarettes a day but drinks very little.

Consultant | On the basis of that history, what do you think is the most important current problem?

Student | Uncontrolled hypertension.

Consultant | How can you make a diagnosis like that from the history he has given?

Student | I found his blood pressure to be very high when I checked it.

Consultant | Yes, but that is a finding on examination. I did not ask you about your clinical examination but about the history. Can you diagnose high blood pressure on symptoms alone?

Student | He was complaining of dizziness which can be caused by high blood pressure.

Consultant | Dizziness is not a symptom of hypertension itself, but may be due either to associated cerebrovascular disease with vertebrobasilar insufficiency, or may be iatrogenic. Do you know what that word means?

Student	No, I'm sorry.
Consultant	It is from the Greek word *iatros* meaning physician; iatrogenic means 'caused by the physician'. 　How can Mr B. have iatrogenic dizziness?
Student	His blood pressure might fall too low with his hypertension tablets.
Consultant	Are Mr B.'s tablets of the type which can cause excessive hypotension?
Student	I'm not sure.
Consultant	Nifedipine is a peripheral vasodilator and is therefore likely to cause postural hypotension and dizziness when he stands up. He was complaining of unsteadiness on getting out of bed in the morning, so this would fit in with postural hyopotension which is always worse first thing in the morning. Can we return now to my earlier question about symptoms specific to hypertension.
Student	Nose-bleeds can occur in patients with high blood pressure.
Consultant	Yes, nose-bleeds can be caused by hypertension but more often they are due to fragile veins at the entrance to the nose. 　Do you know any other symptoms caused by high blood pressure?
Student	Headache is the most likely symptom.
Consultant	What type of headache does Mr B. have?
Student	I'm sorry, I didn't go into much detail with him about the headache. I think it is just a generalized headache.
Consultant	The most rewarding way of diagnosing the cause of a headache is by an accurate and detailed history of the site, character, timing, modifying factors and associated symptoms. If you haven't decided the likely cause on the basis of these characteristics of the headache, it is highly unlikely that you will get much further either with a clinical examination, or even less, with investigations: in this respect the diagnosis of headache is very much like the diagnosis of chest pain. 　Would you like to ask Mr B. some details about his headache?
Student	Mr B., can you tell us in which part of your head you get your headaches, and what it feels like?
Patient	I can get it over the whole of my head or sometimes just at the top. It feels like a 'weight' on top of my head or sometimes like a dull ache all over.
Student	How long do the headaches usually last?
Patient	They often last all day, and sometimes they seem to go on for days at a time.
Student	Does anything make them better or worse.
Patient	I don't seem to be able to get anything to relieve the headache when it is bad. They only started since I had blood pressure, you know — I wasn't troubled much with headaches before.

Consultant	(To student) What do you make of that?
Student	They could be due to his high blood pressure because he says that he hadn't any headache before.
Consultant	They sound much more like 'tension' headache to me; it is common in hypertensive patients and is usually due to anxiety; it may only start after the patient knows his blood pressure is up — as in Mr B.'s case.
	However, there is a distinctive type of headache which is caused by high blood pressure; this is a throbbing occipital headache usually worse either in the middle of the night or first thing in the morning, and may be aggravated by straining.
	Can you think of any other important condition if an elderly male patient suddenly starts to complain of headache, especially in the temporal area?
Student	Do you mean temporal arteritis?
Consultant	That's right. Why is it an important diagnosis to make?
Student	It can cause blindness because it can lead to optic atrophy.
Consultant	Yes, and it can be prevented if high-dose steroid treatment is started right away.
	What is the most important diagnostic test in temporal arteritis?
Student	A high ESR.
Consultant	A high ESR is very frequent though not invariable. It is not the most important test — this is a biopsy of the temporal artery for evidence of arteritis.
	To return to Mr B., what would you say are the first two decisions to make in a patient with hypertension?
Student	How high the blood pressure is and what treatment to give.
Consultant	I agree that those are important but not what I had in mind.
	The first thing to consider is whether the blood pressure is primary (or essential) or secondary to some other underlying condition, particularly if it is a remediable condition. The second important consideration is whether there is any evidence of target organ damage as a result of the blood pressure.
	Do you think that the history can provide you with any information on these two points?
Student	He has a family history of hypertension.
Consultant	What is the relevance of that point?
Student	It suggests essential hypertension which runs in families.
Consultant	Good. That is the most helpful point in diagnosing essential hypertension, a positive family history.
	What about secondary hypertension — what particular factors in the history are relevant?

Student	If there is a past history of kidney disease or if there are any current urinary symptoms.
Consultant	That's right — kidney disease is the commonest cause of secondary hypertension, particularly chronic pyelonephritis. So you may get a past history of recurrent urinary tract infection or current symptoms of frequency and dysuria. Can you think of any other symptoms which might suggest other causes of secondary hypertension?
Student	You might get symptoms of phaeochromocytoma.
Consultant	Which are . . .?
Student	Paroxysmal headache is the most frequent symptom but you can also have palpitations and tremor.
Consultant	That's right. These symptoms are due to the excessive release of nor-adrenaline and/or adrenaline, and can therefore include paroxysmal, or even sustained, headache, palpitations, sweating, trembling and symptoms of anxiety and apprehension. Phaeochromocytoma is a very rare cause of hypertension. What do you know of Conn's* syndrome?
Student	It is caused by a tumour of the adrenal gland and it leads to hyperaldosteronism.
Consultant	What symptoms does it cause?
Student	You can get muscle weakness.
Consultant	What causes the muscle weakness?
Student	It's due to excessive loss of potassium.
Consultant	That's right. The excessive loss of potassium in the urine leads to hypokalaemia which results in muscle weakness. Polyuria and poly-dipsia can also occur due to the impaired concentrating ability of the kidneys. Do you know any other causes of secondary hypertension?
Student	What about renal artery stenosis?
Consultant	That is another cause of secondary hypertension but it can't be diag-nosed on the history — you can tell me later how you would diagnose it. The only other conditions to mention as causes of secondary hyperten-sion are Cushing's* syndrome and coarctation of the aorta. Now let us turn our thoughts to target organ damage as a result of the high blood pressure. What target organs do we have in mind?
Student	The heart is the most obvious one.
Consultant	Any others?

* J.W. Conn is a contemporary American physician born in 1907.
* H.W. Cushing (1869–1939) was an American neurosurgeon.

Student	The arteries I suppose.
Consultant	Hypertension does lead to arterial damage in the form of atherosclerois, but the arteries are not usually specified as target organs. The other organs likely to be affected are the brain and the kidneys. Does Mr B. have any symptoms of target organ damage?
Student	He has angina which indicates that his coronary arteries are affected.
Consultant	What do you think are the factors which cause this damage to Mr B.'s arteries?
Student	The most important factor is the hypertension.
Consultant	Are there any other relevant factors in Mr B.'s history — let's ask Mr B. himself. Mr B., is there anything you can think of which might have helped to cause your heart problem?
Pt. ~~Student~~	I suppose you mean my smoking. I know it's bad for my heart and I've tried to give it up a few times — my wife is always getting on to me about it but it's no good.
Consultant	I would think that the smoking is likely to be the major factor causing the coronary artery disease in Mr B. because, as far as we know, he has only had hypertension for the last two years. What other cardiac complications can occur as a result of hypertension, apart from angina?
Student	You can get heart failure.
Consultant	Yes, left ventricular failure is an important complication of hypertension. Does Mr B. have any symptoms to suggest left ventricular failure?
Student	He becomes breathless on exertion.
Consultant	That is the earliest manifestation of left ventricular failure. How would the breathlessness progress if he remained untreated?
Student	It would get progressively worse so that eventually he would end up breathless at rest.
Consultant	What would be the most serious type of breathlessness he could have?
Student	Paroxysmal nocturnal dyspnoea due to pulmonary oedema.
Consultant	When that occurs the prognosis is very grave. Let's turn to another target organ — the kidney. What symptoms might you get?
Student	You could get dysuria.
Consultant	No, that is only evidence of urinary tract infection. The end result of renal damage by hypertension is renal failure. What symptoms do you get with this?
Student	Hiccups.
Consultant	This is always mentioned first but it is not so common in practice in my

experience, and there are other important symptoms like polyuria and polydipsia, pruritus, twitching, bleeding, diarrhoea and, in the most severe cases of uraemia, drowsiness and coma.

We are now left with the third important target organ which can be affected by hypertension, the brain. Has Mr B. any symptoms of hypertensive brain damage?

Student	He had a slight stroke a year ago.
Consultant	His stroke only lasted 24 hours. We usually have another name for a transient stroke of this kind.
Student	It could be a transient ischaemic attack.
Consultant	That's right, though usually transient ischaemic attacks last less than 24 hours, often no more than a few minutes. If Mr B. had a transient ischaemic attack, what would you think is the likely cause?
Student	A cerebral embolus.
Consultant	Where would a cerebral embolus originate?
Student	The carotid arteries in the neck.
Consultant	Yes, this is the commonest site, and I hope you will refer to it in your examination findings. Any other sites?
Student	The leg veins.
Consultant	No — thrombosis in the leg veins leads to a pulmonary embolus. A blood clot can't get through to the systemic circulation and the brain unless there is an atrial or interventricular septal defect causing a right-to-left shunt, which is a very rare condition in an elderly hypertensive patient. The heart is the other main source of cerebral emboli — what cardiac conditions can cause this?
Student	Atrial fibrillation is the one I've come across most.
Consultant	That is the commonest cardiac cause of cerebral emboli. Mr B. was complaining of palpitations so this should be kept in mind. Do you know any other cardiac cause of emboli?
Student	It can occur in a myocardial infarction.
Consultant	Do you know how?
Student	You can get a blood clot forming in the ventricle over the site of the infarct.
Consultant	What other cardiac causes?
Student	Rheumatic heart disease.
Consultant	That was the commonest cause when I was a student. Do you know why you can get emboli in this condition?
Student	I think it's due to blood clot forming on the diseased valve.

Consultant	That is one reason but there is a much more common cause.
Student	I'm not sure which you mean.
Consultant	The most important predisposing factor for embolization in rheumatic heart disease is the frequency of associated atrial fibrillation. Do you know any other cardiac causes?
Student	No, I don't think so.
Consultant	There are one or two other rare causes like mitral valve prolapse and left atrial myxoma. Let's return to Mr B.'s symptoms. He mentioned excessive tiredness — what do you think the cause is? Could it be iatrogenic?
Student	I don't really know.
Consultant	Tiredness is a common side-effect of a number of drugs used in treating hypertension, especially beta-blockers and methyldopa. He is having nifedipine for his blood pressure and this is not usually associated with excessive fatigue. A complaint of 'tiredness all the time' in my experience, usually suggests a psychological origin.

Now, at this stage we should try to summarize our conclusions on the diagnosis which we have obtained from the history:

HISTORY

- Mr B. has a two-year history of hypertension which is currently being treated with nifedipine
- the family history of hypertension suggests that his hypertension is essential
- there are no symptoms to suggest an underlying renal or endocrine cause for the hypertension
- the headaches are likely to be 'tension' headaches and are not related directly to the high blood pressure
- the postural dizziness is probably due to the effects of the nifedipine which is a peripheral vasodilator
- the angina indicates associated coronary artery disease which is probably due mainly to his smoking, as well as the hypertension
- the breathlessness suggests early left ventricular failure which is likely to be due to a combination of coronary artery disease and target organ damage from the hypertension
- Mr B. had a transient ischaemic attack a year ago and we wonder if this might have been the result of a cerebral embolus from the carotid arteries in the neck or due to atrial fibrillation in view of the history of palpitations

---

Consultant	Now can we turn to your examination findings, and can I suggest that you try to present a problem-orientated examination, which means that

your findings are related to the diagnoses suggested by the history, and not based on a routine general examination such as most students seem taught to do.

Student His general condition is good, he is not breathless or cyanosed, he isn't anaemic and has no enlarged glands.

Consultant Do you think the anaemia and enlarged glands are relevant to his present problems?

Student Probably not.

Consultant So why mention them? This is what I suggested you should not do — adopt a general presentation in the examination findings. His problems indicated by the history are hypertension, coronary artery disease and cerebrovascular disease; I would like you to try to relate your findings to these conditions (Figure 3.1).

Student I'm sorry. I'll start again with the cardiovascular system. His pulse was 84/min and regular. The blood pressure was 170/115 in both arms, the apex beat seemed normal and the heart sounds were normal with no murmurs.

Consultant Did you record the blood pressure lying in bed or standing up?

Student I checked it with Mr B. in bed.

Consultant Do you think it important to check it standing up as well?

Student Yes, I should have done that.

Consultant It is important because he is being treated with a peripheral vasodilator, nifedipine, and we are wondering whether his dizziness could be due to postural hypotension as a result of this treatment. Also the standing blood pressure will tell us whether blood pressure control is satisfactory when he is up and about.

Would you like to check it now?

The student checks Mr B.'s blood pressure both standing and lying; he finds 175/115 (lying) and 115/55 (standing). Mr B. also complains of feeling dizzy when he stands up.

Consultant Before I ask you to comment on these readings, I'd like to ask you whether you used phase 4 of the Korotkov* sounds (the muffling of the sounds) to record your diastolic pressure, or phase 5 (the complete disappearance of the sounds).

Student We're taught to use phase 4.

Consultant So was I when I was a student. The 5th phase gives a more accurate

---

* N.G. Korotkov was a Russian surgeon born in 1876 who introduced auscultatory measurement of blood pressure in 1905.

measurement of the diastolic pressure when compared with a direct intra-arterial recording. Perhaps the best way to resolve this dilemma is to record both 4th and 5th phase readings in all patients.

Now, would you like to comment on your own readings?

Student

There is no doubt about the postural hypotension and this is what makes him dizzy when he stands up.

Consultant

I agree. He seems very sensitive to the nifedipine and I think his treatment will therefore need to be changed.

You mentioned in your examination that Mr B.'s heart sounds were normal. What abnormality would you expect to find in a patient with hypertension?

Student

He might have a murmur.

Consultant

Murmurs are not a common finding in hypertensive patients except in one important but relatively rare condition — do you know what it is?

Student

I'm not sure.

Consultant

Coarctation of the aorta. You can get a rough mid-systolic murmur along the left sternal border; you can also hear it at the back over the left scapula.

What other findings might you get in coarctation?

Student

The femoral pulses will be absent.

Consultant

That's right. Don't forget also about abnormal scapular pulsation. Co-arctation is an important condition to keep in mind, especially in the young hypertensive, because it is completely reversible by operation.

What other abnormal findings might you get on auscultation in a hypertensive patient?

Student

A gallop rhythm.

Consultant

Good. A gallop rhythm is heard when there is an additional heart sound; it may be either a presystolic gallop due to a 4th, or atrial, heart sound, or a protodiastolic gallop due to a 3rd heart sound. An atrial gallop indicates either left ventricular strain or left ventricular failure; a protodiastolic gallop means heart failure, either left or right, when it occurs in an older patient — it can occur normally in a young healthy person.

If you thought that the gallop rhythm was due to left ventricular failure, what other confirmatory signs might you look for?

Student

Crepitations in the lungs.

Consultant

That's right. In left ventricular failure you hear fine crepitations which tend to occur in 'showers'.

Do you know the mechanism of the crepitations?

Student

They are due to pulmonary congestion.

Consultant

The other important sign in left ventricular failure is of course breathlessness.

	Is there any other auscultatory sign in the heart which is relevant in a hypertensive patient?
Student	I can't think of any more.
Consultant	What about the intensity of the aortic 2nd sound at the base of the heart.
Student	I suppose that it would be loud.
Consultant	What would be the clinical significance of a loud 2nd sound at the aortic area?
Student	Is it related to the height of the blood pressure?
Consultant	Yes, that is true — the higher the blood pressure the louder the sound, but the other significant fact that it tells us is that the hypertension is likely to be long-standing. What was Mr B.'s aortic 2nd sound like?
Student	I must admit that I didn't pay much attention to it because I hadn't realized that it was so significant.
Consultant	Would you like to listen again now?

The student listens carefully to Mr B.'s heart and decides that the aortic 2nd sound is louder than normal. The consultant also listens and agrees with him.

Consultant	Mr B.'s loud 2nd sound would suggest to me that his hypertension was probably present a lot longer than two years. Apart from the heart and lungs, did you find anything on examination?
Student	I couldn't find any abdominal tenderness to suggest any recurrence of his ulcer. There were no abdominal masses.
Consultant	What abdominal masses were you looking for?
Student	An enlarged liver or spleen.
Consultant	Is that relevant in a hypertensive patient?
Student	I suppose not.
Consultant	There is another abdominal organ which could be relevant in a hypertensive patient.
Student	He didn't have any renal enlargement.
Consultant	That's better. What might cause renal enlargement in a hypertensive patient?
Student	He could have polycystic disease.
Consultant	Right, though it is a rare condition. Don't forget unilateral renal disease like hydronephrosis can also lead to hypertension associated with a large kidney. Did you look for anything else in the abdomen?
Student	His femoral pulses were normal.
Consultant	Good. Anything else?

Student	I can't think of any other relevant findings.
Consultant	You should always listen for a systolic murmur over the renal arteries in hypertensive patients — this would suggest renal artery stenosis which, like coarctation, is a potentially reversible cause of the hypertension. Would you like to tell us about his nervous system?
Student	I couldn't find any abnormality, and in particular, there were no residual signs from his previous stroke.
Consultant	Can you tell us about his fundi?
Student	I could only get a limited view because his pupils were small; I thought they were normal.
Consultant	You should always ask to have the pupils dilated to have a good look at the fundi in a hypertensive patient, but be careful you don't do this if there is any possibility of glaucoma, particularly in an elderly patient. What changes might occur in the fundi of a hypertensive patient?
Student	Arterio-venous nipping.
Consultant	Yes, that is regarded as grade II hypertensive retinopathy: grade I is arteriolar narrowing and irregularity. When do you get grades III and IV?
Student	In malignant hypertension.
Consultant	What other changes do you get in grades III and IV in malignant hypertension?
Student	Haemorrhages and exudates.
Consultant	The haemorrhages are in the superficial layers of the retina and therefore they appear flame-shaped: the exudates are also superficial and they look fluffy, like 'cotton wool'. There is one other very important finding in the fundi in malignant hypertension — do you know what it is?
Student	You get papilloedema.
Consultant	That's right. Now I think we will ask sister if she would be good enough to put some tropicamide drops into Mr B.'s eyes to dilate his pupils and then you could tell us what you can see.
	When the pupils are adequately dilated the student reports that he can see definite arterio-venous nipping in both fundi, but he could not see any haemorrhages or exudates and he did not think there was any papilloedema.
Consultant	I agree with your findings though I would also add that there is narrowing and irregularity of the arterioles. How would you grade Mr B.'s retinopathy?
Student	I would call it Grade II.
Consultant	That is correct. Now we have so far considered the main target organs of the hyper-

	tension, the heart, the brain and the kidneys. Would you like to let us have your comments now about Mr B.'s arteries?
Student	I checked his foot pulses; I could feel the posterior tibial pulses on both sides but neither dorsalis pedis.
Consultant	That shows there is some peripheral arterial disease though he doesn't complain of claudication. Did you check any other arteries?
Student	Only the radial pulse.
Consultant	Was the radial artery thickened?
Student	I didn't think so.
Consultant	If you are looking for atherosclerosis you should also check for thickening, and sometimes tortuosity, of the radial artery and the brachial artery — a condition called a locomotor brachial artery. Other useful indications of atherosclerosis are systolic murmurs over the carotid and femoral arteries, as well as over the abdominal aorta. There is one other important clue to atherosclerosis, particularly premature atherosclerosis — do you know what this is?
Student	I'm not sure.
Consultant	You would see it in the patient's eyes.
Student	Oh, you mean xanthelasma.
Consultant	That's one sign but there is another important sign in the eyes themselves.
Student	Do you mean an arcus senilis?
Consultant	I mean a premature arcus senilis in a young patient. Together with xanthelasma, the arcus senilis suggests hypercholesterolaemia and the consequent likelihood of premature atherosclerosis, if you have these signs in a young patient — an arcus senilis would be less relevant in an older patient like Mr B. Is there anything else you want to tell us about Mr B.'s examination?
Student	No, I don't think so apart from mentioning that he still has bad varicose veins in both legs but there is no sign of acute thrombophlebitis.
Consultant	I think we should now try to summarize the relevant findings in the examination and indicate the conclusion we derive from them. Now, I think we should consider the investigation of Mr B.'s problems. What tests do you think we need?
Student	I would do a full blood count first.
Consultant	Why do you want a blood count?
Student	All hospital patients have a routine blood count.
Consultant	Regrettably, that is usually the case — in my view, a routine blood count is an unnecessary practice and rarely gives much help in managing patients. Let's try to suggest tests that are relevant to Mr B.'s problems.

EXAMINATION

- we have confirmed that Mr B. has hypertension
- he has definite postural hypotension which was associated with dizziness
- there were no abnormal signs to suggest either a renal or endocrine cause for the hypertension nor was there any evidence of coarctation of the aorta
- there was no dyspnoea, gallop rhythm or pulmonary crepitations to indicate left ventricular failure
- the absence of the dorsalis pedis pulses in both feet indicates peripheral vascular disease
- the fundi show grade II hypertensive retinopathy thus confirming arteriosclerosi

Student	Can we start with the blood urea and serum electrolytes?
Consultant	I would agree that the blood urea is relevant in hypertension. In what way might it help?
Student	It would indicate any underlying renal disease.
Consultant	Yes, this may be relevant in the aetiology of the hypertension. What else might it tell you?
Student	It will show whether there is any renal failure.
Consultant	In other words, it will also indicate the effect of the hypertension on the target organ, the kidney. What about the electrolytes — do you need to know them all or is there any particularly important one in hypertension?
Student	The serum potassium is the most important electrolyte.
Consultant	Why do you think that?
Student	It would help us to pick up Conn's syndrome.
Consultant	Yes, we talked about primary hyperaldosteronism or Conn's syndrome earlier when we discussed the history. What other tests help you to diagnose Conn's syndrome?
Student	You could measure the aldosterone level in the blood.
Consultant	That is if you have facilities available for this test which is most unlikely in the ordinary district general hospital like this one. The other important test if you suspect hyperaldosteronism is to measure the plasma renin level — this would be low in primary hyperaldosteronism due to Conn's syndrome, and high in secondary hyperaldosteronism due to malignant hypertension or renal artery stenosis. Now, to return to Mr B.'s blood urea and serum electrolyte results, here are the figures (page 65). What do you make of them?

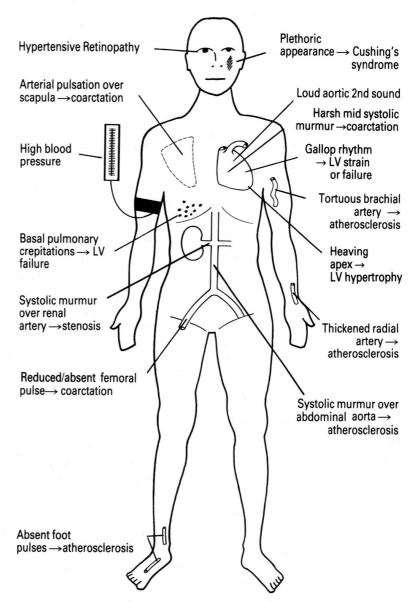

Figure 3.1 Possible signs in a hypertensive patient.

		Normal range
Blood urea	8.2 mmol/L	3.3– 6.6
Serum creatinine	151 μmol/L	60–100
Sodium	136 mmol/L	135–145
Potassium	4.2 mmol/L	3.3– 5.5
Chloride	99 mmol/L	95–105
Bicarbonate	23 mmol/L	22–32

Student	It shows that he is mildly uraemic with a raised blood urea and serum creatinine level, but there is no hypokalaemia to suggest hyperaldosteronism and the other electrolytes seem OK.
Consultant	I would agree with that analysis. I would think the mild uraemia is the result of target organ damage to the kidneys. What other tests do we want in Mr B.?
Student	A chest X-ray.
Consultant	What would you look for in the chest X-ray?
Student	I would look for cardiac enlargement.
Consultant	The importance of cardiomegaly is that it indicates a more adverse prognosis in a hypertensive patient. You have already told us in your examination that you found no clinical evidence of cardiac enlargement, as indicated by a normal apex beat, and Mr B.'s X-ray confirms that he has no significant cardiomegaly. However, I do have an X-ray of another patient with substantial left ventricular enlargement as a result of hypertension and I thought you would like to see it; it is typical of what we call a 'boot-shaped' heart (Figure 3.2).
Consultant	Does the chest X-ray help us in any other way in a hypertensive patient?
Student	It may show left ventricular failure.
Consultant	That's true; it may show the early indications of left ventricular failure when there are not yet any clinical signs on examination. Do you know what the early radiological sign is?
Student	I don't think so.
Consultant	The earliest sign of left ventricular failure in the chest X-ray is upper lobe venous congestion. Is there any other important information in the chest X-ray in hypertension?
Student	I can't think of anything else.
Consultant	What about coarctation of the aorta?

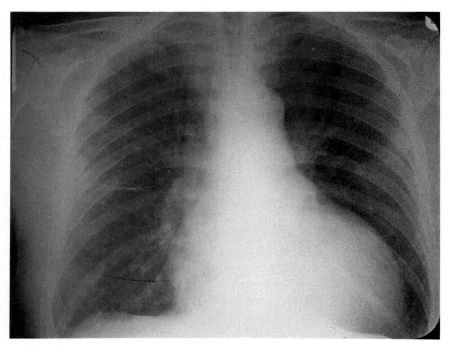

Figure 3.2   Chest X-ray showing a 'boot-shaped' heart in a patient with left ventricular enlargement due to hypertension.

Student	I'm sorry, I forgot about that. You can get notching of the ribs.
Consultant	What causes the notching?
Student	I think it's something to do with the collateral circulation that you get in this condition.
Consultant	That's right. Branches of the subclavian artery above the constriction in the aorta bypass the obstruction by anastomosing with the intercostal arteries and the internal mammary arteries to link up with the aorta below the obstruction. I thought you might like to see this X-ray which shows beautiful notching in another patient I had with a coarctation (Figure 3.3).
Consultant	Do you want any other tests for Mr B.?
Student	I think he should have an ECG.
Consultant	In what way would it help our management of Mr B.?
Student	It might tell us whether he had any ischaemia.
Consultant	Don't you know that already — didn't you tell us that Mr B. had angina?
Student	Well, yes we do know he has ischaemia from the history but won't the ECG tell us how bad it is.

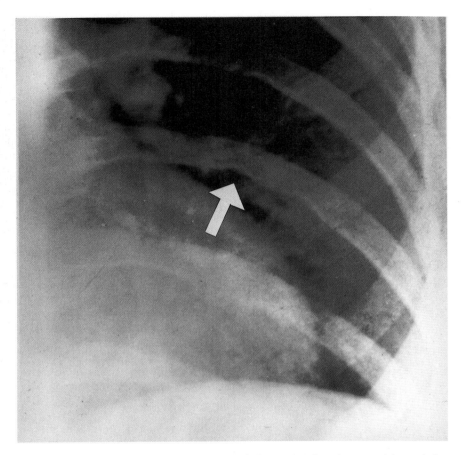

Figure 3.3 Chest X-ray in coarctation of the aorta showing notching of the lower margins of the ribs (arrowed) due to erosion by the enlarged intercostal arteries helping the circulation to bypass the constriction in the aorta.

Consultant	Now, you're asking a different — and I might say a more relevant — question of the ECG. If the ECG does show ischaemic damage, say a previous myocardial infarction, what help would it be to you in managing Mr B.'s problems?
Student	I'm not really sure.
Consultant	The main significance of such an ECG finding is in assessing prognosis — it would obviously suggest a more adverse prognosis.
	There is perhaps a more important abnormality that we should look for in the ECG of a hypertensive patient, isn't there?
Student	Is it to see if left ventricular hypertrophy is present?
Consultant	That's right, and the importance of this — like cardiac enlargement on

chest X-ray — it indicates a more unfavourable prognosis; even more so if there is left ventricular strain.

Fortunately, Mr B.'s ECG doesn't show any left ventricular hypertrophy or strain, but I do have another patient's ECG to show you with these abnormalities on it (Figure 3.4).

Any other tests?

Student	We could check his urine for protein.
Consultant	Proteinuria would indicate renal damage and would occur especially in malignant hypertension. What else might you look for in the urine if you suspected malignant hypertension?
Student	You might find blood in the urine.
Consultant	That's right, but it is usually detectable only on microscopy. What about casts in the urine?
Student	I don't really know much about casts.
Consultant	No, no-one seems to bother much about coasts these days. When I was a student, granular casts seen on microscopy of the urine were regarded as an important sign of renal damage, especially from chronic nephritis. Are there any other renal tests which you think could be useful?
Student	An intravenous pyelogram.
Consultant	A routine IVP is not usually necessary in hypertensive patients. When do you think it would be indicated?
Student	If you suspect kidney disease.
Consultant	That's right, it would be useful then. It is also indicated in all young hypertensive patients because they have a higher incidence of secondary hypertension, often of renal origin like chronic pyelonephritis or polycystic disease (Figure 3.5). Another useful function of the IVP would be to show renal artery stenosis, when the dye excretion is delayed and more concentrated in the affected kidney. Are there any other relevant tests you would like?
Student	What about urinary catecholamines for phaeochromocytoma?
Consultant	That's a very rare condition. I think it's only worth investigating if the patient has any suggestive symptoms, like . . .
Student	Paroxysmal headache.
Consultant	It may also be sustained headache. Other symptoms due to excess catecholamines in the blood include palpitations, sweating and trembling. How would you confirm the diagnosis?
Student	Would an IVP help?
Consultant	Only if there were a large adrenal tumour distorting the kidney. The best test for phaeochromocytoma nowadays is a CT scan. Can you think of any other useful X-rays in a hypertensive patient?

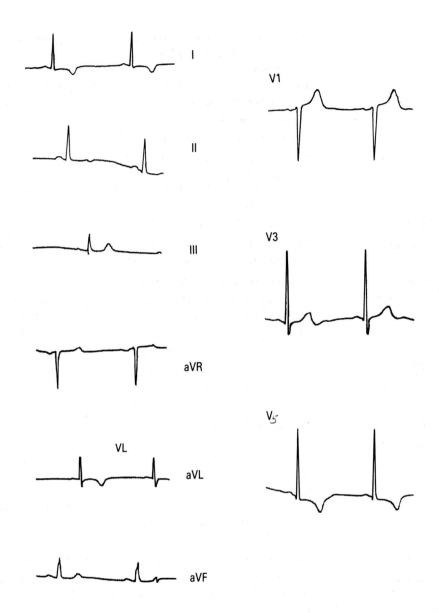

Figure 3.4 Electrocardiogram showing left ventricular hypertrophy (deep S in V1 and tall R in V5) and associated strain (ST depression with T inversion in V5).

Student	I don't think so.
Consultant	A renal arteriogram is necessary if you suspect renal artery stenosis.
	Now, I would like to spend a little time briefly considering the treatment of hypertension.
	Mr B. is having nifedipine for his blood pressure; how does this work?

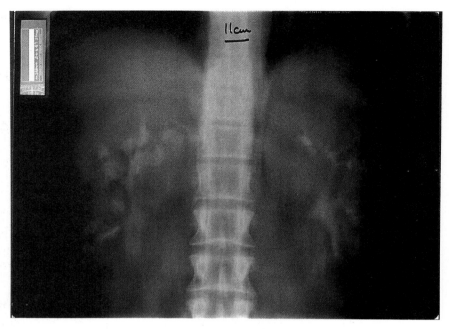

Figure 3.5 Intravenous pyelogram in a patient with polycystic disease affecting the kidneys showing distortion of the calyces by large renal cysts.

Student	Nifedipine is a calcium antagonist and it works by dilating the peripheral arteries.
Consultant	That is correct and it accounts of course for Mr B.'s postural dizziness when he stands up and his blood pressure falls too much. Peripheral vasodilators should always be used with great caution for this reason in elderly hypertensive patients with cerebral arteriosclerosis. You can also see why it is important to check the standing blood pressure if you are using this type of drug. Do you know any other side-effects of nifedipine?
Student	You can get throbbing headache.
Consultant	And facial flushing. Any others?
Student	Swelling of the ankles.
Consultant	That's fairly common. Palpitations due to reflex tachycardia can also be a problem sometimes and may need a beta-blocker. There are other calcium antagonists used for hypertension as well, like verapamil which is quite an effective drug, though it is prone to cause constipation in some patients. What other drugs would you consider for treating hypertension?
Student	Thiazides are used a lot.

Consultant	Thiazides are only mild hypotensive agents and do have a number of disadvantages, don't they?
Student	They can cause hyperglycaemia and gout.
Consultant	That's right and other side-effects include impotence and an increase in blood lipids.
Student	What about hypokalaemia?
Consultant	It is rarely a problem with the thiazides in my experience, unlike the use of loop diuretics like frusemide. Thiazides may be of value in treating mild hypertension especially in older patients but I rarely use them myself. What other hypotensive drugs do you know?
Student	Beta-blockers are in widespread use.
Consultant	Yes, beta-blockers are effective hypotensive agents and are specially useful if there is associated angina. They, too, have their disadvantages; would you like to mention some?
Student	They can cause asthma.
Consultant	Bronchoconstriction is a significant side-effect and these drugs must be avoided as far as possible in any patients with an airway problem like chronic bronchitis or asthma — this is quite common here in Barnsley. This effect is less marked if you use a cardio-selective beta-blocker like atenolol rather than a non-selective one like propranolol. What other side-effects are there with beta-blockers?
Student	They can reduce the peripheral circulation.
Consultant	Therefore you would not use them in patients with intermittent claudication. Any others?
Student	I can't think of any more.
Consultant	An important side-effect is a depressant effect on myocardial function, so you would be careful in a patient with heart failure. Like the thiazides, beta-blockers can also increase blood lipids and sometimes cause impotence. Another side-effect which, in my experience is a lot more common than most doctors realize, is debilitating fatigue. What is the newest type of drug to be introduced for hypertension?
Student	Is it angiotensin-converting enzyme inhibitors (ACEI)?
Consultant	That's right. Do you know how they work?
Student	They reduce the blood level of angiotensin.
Consultant	And do you know what the normal action of circulating angiotensin is?
Student	It increases the blood pressure by peripheral vasoconstriction.
Consultant	Good. There is one other physiological function of angiotensin, isn't there?

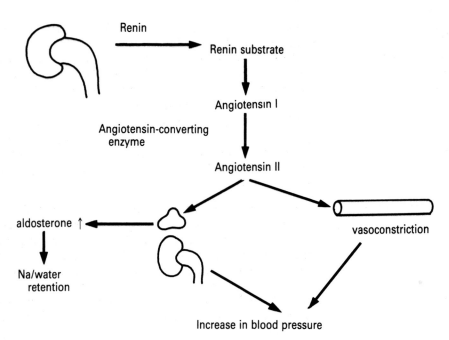

Figure 3.6   Renin/angiotensin/ aldosterone system.

Student	I'm not sure.
Consultant	It stimulates the adrenal gland to secrete aldosterone (Figure 3.6).
	An ACEI acts in hypertension mainly by reducing circulating angiotensin and therefore allowing peripheral vasodilation to occur. The inhibition of aldosterone production by the ACEI is of more value in treating heart failure.
	I find the ACEIs very useful in treating hypertension and I am using them increasingly now. They have few side-effects when used carefully and you must always start with a low dose to pick up those few patients who are unduly sensitive and react with a severe fall in standing blood pressure. The initial alarm about the renal toxic effects and depression of the bone marrow was fortunately not borne out by subsequent experience, provided you are careful with the size of the dose and avoid treating patients with renal impairment at the start.
	I just want to finish now by asking you your views on whether we should treat mild hypertension — say a pressure above 160/95 in asymptomatic people?
Student	I don't really know the answer.
Consultant	Do you know what benefits the control of hypertension is supposed to achieve.
Student	It reduces strokes and heart failure.

Consultant
That's right but unfortunately it doesn't do much for the prevention of coronary disease.

There is good evidence that control of even mild hypertension can prevent strokes in a few patients but a lot of other patients will be treated unnecessarily, with the anxiety that may induce as well as having uncomfortable side-effects.

What we need therefore are some simple guidelines on selecting the patients with mild hypertension who may be at increased risk of complications of the raised blood pressure. Have you any ideas?

Student
The patient would be at more risk if he had any of the other risk factors like smoking.

Consultant
That is an important point. Smoking is the main hazard but other risk factors would include a high blood cholesterol, diabetes, obesity and — very important — a bad family history of hypertension or *premature* ischaemic heart disease; also don't forget the use of the contraceptive pill in women especially if they are smokers as well.

There is one other important consideration which would suggest the need for treatment in an asymptomatic patient with mild blood pressure: we discussed this earlier when we considered the harmful effects of hypertension.

OUTCOME

The nifedipine was stopped because of the postural hypotension, and the standing blood pressure rose to 160/110 and the dizziness disappeared.

It was decided to avoid using any other peripheral vasodilator because of the possibility of recurrence of the postural hypotension. Beta-blockers were contraindicated because of the chronic bronchitis. Accordingly, he was treated with methyldopa, starting with 125 mg tds, then increasing to 250 mg tds after a few days. On this régime he seemed quite happy with no recurrence of his dizziness though there was still a slight postural drop of blood pressure from 165/100 (lying) to 155/95 (standing).

One additional advantage of using methyldopa in Mr B. was that it was likely to have a beneficial effect on his renal blood flow, which is important in view of his mild renal failure.

During a subsequent two-year follow-up in the medical clinic blood pressure control stayed satisfactorily controlled and there were no significant side-effects attributable to the methyldopa. The angina also remained controlled using isosorbide mononitrate 20 mg bd, together with the free prophylactic use of sublingual trinitrin.

Renal function, as indicated by the blood urea and serum creatinine levels, stayed constant over the period of follow-up.

Student   You mean whether there is target organ damage as a result of the hypertension.

Consultant   That's right. X-ray evidence of cardiac enlargement or ECG evidence of left ventricular enlargement would be a spur to starting urgent treatment.

One final and very important point in relation to the diagnosis of mild hypertension: the diagnosis should not be made until at least three blood pressure measurements are made at not less than monthly intervals, because a large number of these individuals will settle down to normal blood pressure levels without any treatment at all.

LEARNING POINTS

Difference between hypertensive and 'tension' headache

	Hypertension	*'Tension' headache*
Type	throbbing	pressure weight tight band other bizarre descriptions
Site	occipital	vertex 'all over'
Timing	night early morning	any time worse with stress
Duration	few hours	hours, days

Causes of hypertension

- primary (essential) — 90 to 95%
- secondary-renal
        chronic pyelonephritis
        chronic glomerulonephritis
        hydronephrosis
        polycystic disease
        renal artery stenosis
    -adrenal
        Conn's syndrome
        phaeochromocytoma
        Cushing's disease
    -coarctation of the aorta

Symptoms of phaeochromocytoma

- paroxysmal or sustained throbbing headache
- palpitations
- excessive sweating
- tremor
- feelings of hunger and apprehension
- angina — occasionally

Target organ damage as a result of hypertension

- heart
    enlargement
    ischaemia — angina/infarction
    left ventricular failure
- brain
    haemorrhagic stroke
    thrombotic stroke — less directly related

- kidneys
  - renal failure
- arteries
  - peripheral → intermittent claudication
  - fundi → retinopathy
  - mesenteric → mesenteric 'angina'
  - carotid → transient ischaemic attacks

Causes of cerebral emboli

carotid atheroma in the neck
cardiac
- atrial fibrillation
- valvular heart disease
  - rheumatic
  - infective endocarditis
  - prosthesis
  - mitral valve prolapse
- mural thrombus (myocardial infarction)
- left atrial myxoma

Hypertensive retinopathy

Grade I
  - arteriolar irregularity
  - normal veins
Grade II
  - grade I changes
  - arterio-venous nipping
Grade III
  - grade II changes
  - fluffy 'cotton wool' exudates
  - flame-shaped haemorrhages
Grade IV
  - grade III changes
  - venous distension
  - papilloedema

Diagnostic triad in left ventricular failure

- breathlessness
- gallop rhythm
- pulmonary crepitations

Side-effects of calcium antagonists

nifedipine
- headache
- flushing
- palpitations
- ankle swelling

verapamil
- constipation
- depression of myocardial contractility
- impaired a–v conduction

both
- postural hypotension with dizziness

Side-effects of thiazides

- hyperglycaemia (exacerbation of diabetes)
- gout
- impotence
- increase in blood lipids
- hypokalaemia (mild and occasional only)

Side-effects of beta-blockers

- bronchospasm — so avoid in obstructive lung disease
- reduced peripheral circulation — so avoid in claudication and Raynaud's* syndrome
- masking of hypoglycaemia — so use with care in diabetics
- impotence — caution in young sexually-active men
- increase in blood lipids — clinical significance as yet not clear

Indications for treatment of mild hypertension

- bad family history
  hypertension or premature heart disease
  ischaemic heart disease
- target organ damage
  heart
    angina
    heart failure
    enlargement (X-ray, ECG)
  brain
    previous haemorrhagic stroke

* M. Raynaud (1834–1881) was a French physician who described his disease in a thesis submitted to the medical school in Paris. He worked at the famous Hotel Dieu Hospital and was made an officer of the Légion d'honneur in 1871.

           kidneys
              raised blood urea

- associated risk factors
           smoking
           hypercholesterolaemia
           diabetes
           contraceptive pill in women

4

Swelling of the legs

Student   The history here is very short. Mrs J.C. is 43 years old. She was apparently quite well until a few weeks ago when she noticed that her feet were starting to swell. At the same time she found that she was tiring more easily than usual so that she was unable to do her housework. Her feet have become more swollen since the onset so that now she has difficulty in getting her shoes on and also finds that her legs feel 'heavy' when she walks. There is really very little else to add in the history; she has always been fit and is very worried now as to why her feet are so swollen.

Consultant   That is certainly a brief history, albeit a very interesting one — an acute onset of progressive swelling of the feet in an apparently fit woman. Obviously we will need to look for more specific information from the history to try to get some clue as to possible causes of Mrs C.'s problem. How are you going to approach this and I hope you won't mind my stressing that what we are concerned with at the moment is the history not the examination or any tests that may be required later.

Student   I've already mentioned that there was no relevant past history.

Consultant   Like what?

Student   Any heart trouble or any kidney trouble.

Consultant   I'm glad that you are thinking along the right lines. Cardiac oedema and renal oedema are certainly two of the most important causes of swelling of the feet. Incidentally, when you said that there was no previous history of heart disease I hope that you have included rheumatic fever and chorea.

Student   Yes, I did ask specifically about both of those conditions.

Consultant   Can you suggest any other possible cause of bilateral swelling of the legs that we ought to keep in mind?

Student   Do you mean oedema due to varicose veins?

Consultant   No, that's not what I had in mind but it's not a bad suggestion. You can get stasis oedema from varicose veins and it could affect both legs but it usually tends to be asymmetrical. You have mentioned the heart and the kidneys as possible causes of oedema; is there any other major organ that is involved in maintaining fluid balance?

Student   You mean the liver.

Consultant   How is the liver concerned with fluid balance?

Student   It is responsible for the synthesis of albumin which is necessary to maintain the osmotic pressure of the blood.

Consultant   Very good! In hepatic disease the production of albumin is reduced and as a result the plasma osmotic pressure falls and fluid escapes from the circulation leading to oedema. There is one other important physiological change that occurs in liver disease which also contributes to the development of oedema — do you know what it is?

Student   No, I'm sorry.

Consultant   It's connected with the excessive blood levels of a certain hormone . . .

Student   Aldosterone?

Consultant   Aldosterone production is increased in severe liver disease which causes sodium and fluid retention.
                 Has Mrs C. had any liver problems in the past?

Student   I don't think so but I didn't ask her specifically. Mrs C., have you had any trouble with your liver in the past?

Consultant   Not a particularly good way of finding out about liver disease, is it? The patient may not know anything about her liver but she would certainly know whether she has had jaundice or gallstones — those are the sort of questions you should be asking her.

Patient   I think I did have an attack of yellow jaundice when I was about 6 years old but I have never had any trouble with gallstones.

Consultant   Thank you, Mrs C. I doubt if the jaundice at 6 years old had any bearing on her present problem with oedema.
                 Before we leave the possible causes of excessive fluid retention we should not forget that drugs may be responsible — can you suggest any?

Student   Non-steroidal anti-inflammatory drugs.

Consultant   And don't forget that the steroids themselves are potent fluid retainers.
                 There is one other drug used for peptic ulcer treatment which may cause oedema — it's not used so often now. Do you know what it is?

Student   Is it one of the H_2-blockers?

Consultant   No, I'm referring to carbenoxolone.
                 Can you think of any other fluid-retaining drugs? What about in young women?

Student   The contraceptive pill can cause oedema.

Consultant   Yes, any oestrogen preparation can lead to fluid retention. The other group of drugs worth keeping in mind are the vasodilator drugs used in treating hypertension, like nifedipine, hydralazine and minoxidil.

Mrs C., however, has not taken any of these drugs.

Now back to the history. In the light of our comments on the three important causes of leg oedema — heart disease, liver disease and kidney disease; was there anything on enquiry, either negative or positive, that might be relevant?

Student	Well, in relation to her heart, she has not had any angina or breathlessness.
Consultant	If she were breathless, what kind of heart failure would that indicate?
Student	Left ventricular failure.
Consultant	That's right and that is not usually associated with leg oedema unless it is chronic and has led to the development of ...
Student	Right ventricular failure.
Consultant	And it's right ventricular failure which is associated with leg oedema. Breathlessness therefore is not a very helpful symptom in elucidating leg oedema. On the other hand, your comment about angina is relevant as ischaemic heart disease can lead to the development of right ventricular failure though it is not the commonest cause — which is?
Student	Chronic lung disease.
Consultant	This certainly applies to the Barnsley area and many other mining areas in the North. Are there any other relevant points in the history?
Student	With regard to the liver we've already established that she hasn't had gallstones and you thought that her previous jaundice wasn't significant. The other thing to mention is that she drinks very little alcohol.
Consultant	That's a good point since cirrhosis is the commonest type of liver disease to cause oedema. Which professions would you say are at greatest risk of getting alcoholic cirrhosis?
Student	Publicans are the obvious ones.
Consultant	That's right. What others?
Student	I believe our own profession is at high risk.
Consultant	I'm not sure if you mean your profession — medical students — or mine — doctors!
Student	I would say both!
Consultant	I don't think we had better get into an argument about the propensity of the two professions in becoming alcoholics though I have my own views as to who would win — or perhaps lose would be the better way of expressing it! However, I am sure we both agree that Mrs C. does not have this particular problem. Now, let's return to the history, and in particular, whether there were any symptoms to suggest involvement of the other main organ concerned with oedema, the kidney.

Student	I asked her about dysuria but she didn't have any.
Consultant	I would be more interested in polyuria than dysuria.
Student	I'm afraid I didn't ask her about that. Mrs C., have you been passing more urine than usual?
Patient	I have noticed that I have been getting up at night recently to pass water which I haven't ever needed to do before.
Consultan	(To student) What do you think that might signify?
Student	It could mean that she was developing renal failure.
Consultant	That's right. In renal failure the kidneys can't concentrate the urine adequately and so large amounts of dilute urine are passed leading often to nocturia. Incidentally, apart from renal failure, what are the other important causes of polyuria which you should always keep in mind?
Student	Diabetes mellitus.
Consultant	Good, but don't forget diabetes insipidus also but this is of course much rarer that diabetes mellitus. Can you think of any other symptoms of renal failure?
Student	Hiccups.
Consultant	Yes, everyone mentions that one. Any others?
Student	Drowsiness and convulsions.
Consultant	Drowsiness is common but convulsions would only occur in advanced renal failure with a very high blood urea. Anything else?
Student	I believe you can get diarrhoea.
Consultant	Uraemic colitis can occur and cause diarrhoea, but in my experience this is rare though I have dealt with many patients with chronic renal failure. Any other symptoms?
Student	I can't think of any.
Consultant	There are several others: breathlessness due to acidosis (Kussmaul* breathing), twitching, pruritus, spontaneous bleeding due to a combination of platelet disorder and increased capillary permeability, and

---

HISTORY

- Mrs C., a 43-year-old lady, has developed an acute onset of progressive oedema
- there is no past history of rheumatic fever, chorea or cardiac symptoms to suggest a cardiac origin
- although she had transient jaundice in childhood we think this is probably irrelevant
- she does have recent polyuria which might indicate early renal failure and suggests that the oedema could have a renal cause

paraesthesiae due to uraemic peripheral neuropathy. Let us summarize Mrs C.'s history.

Consultant	Now we can proceed with the examination. Before you start to present your findings may I remind you, as I always do at this stage with all students, that the examination should be focused on any signs which may support or exclude the diagnoses you have already considered on the basis of the history — in other words, a problem-orientated examination approach.
	So, what diagnoses are you going to keep in mind?
Student	I shall be thinking of the three main diagnoses of heart failure, kidney disease and liver disease (Figure 4.1).
Consultant	Right, go ahead.
Student	First of all, I was struck by the puffiness around her eyes and I thought this might indicate kidney disease.
Consultant	Very good. Periorbital oedema is an important distinguishing sign in differentiating renal oedema from oedema due to right ventricular failure where periorbital oedema virtually never occurs. Go on.
Student	She looks a bit pale.
Consultant	I agree. Why should that be?
Student	It could be due to anaemia as a result of renal failure.
Consultant	Renal failure is a possible cause, though iron-deficiency is a much more common cause in women of Mrs C.'s age; still we must keep it in mind.
	Would you like to remind us of the mechanism of anaemia in renal failure?
Student	We have already mentioned bleeding.
Consultant	Yes, but Mrs C. has not had any bleeding as far as she knows.
Student	You can get bone marrow depression in uraemia.
Consultant	Do you know why?
Student	I think it's due to a lack of the erythropoietic factor which comes from the kidney and is necessary for normal bone marrow function.
Consultant	Good. It is also suggested that the uraemia itself might have a toxic effect on the marrow. There is one other contributory factor in the anaemia.
Student	I don't know.
Consultant	Increased haemolysis. This is due to an abnormal plasma and not to a red cell abnormality. Let's continue with the examination.
Student	She has marked pitting oedema of the legs up to the knees.

---

* A. Kussmaul (1822–1902) was Professor of Medicine successively at Heidelberg, Erlangen, Freiberg and Strasbourg. He was the first to describe polyarteritis nodosa and was also the first to attempt gastroscopy.

Consultant	Yes, as we can now demonstrate.

The consultant pits Mrs C.'s legs in several sites.

Consultant	Did you notice anything about the speed with which the pitting disappeared?
Student	It seemed to be quite rapid.
Consultant	That's correct. It has been suggested that this may help to distinguish renal oedema from cardiac oedema when the pit stays for a longer time. Have you any idea why this might be?
Student	I don't really know.

Consultant	It may be due to the different mechanisms of oedema in the two conditions.
	  Renal oedema is due to excessive loss of albumin in the urine which reduces the osmotic pressure of the plasma leading to oedema; the pressure relationships at the arterial and venous ends of the capillaries remain normal. In right ventricular failure, however, the oedema is largely due to increased pressure at the venous end of the capillary so that reabsorption of the tissue fluid is impaired — this could lead to a slower resolution of the oedematous pit.
	  Are there any other sites of oedema in Mrs C.?

Student	I wondered whether she might have some ascites.
Consultant	Why did you think that?
Student	Her abdomen seems distended and I thought she had some shifting dullness.
Consultant	I agree, the abdomen is distended, the important thing being that the distension is in the flanks and not central. I would agree also that she has shifting dullness. Did you check for any other signs of fluid?
Student	I tried for a fluid thrill but I wasn't convinced.
Consultant	The fluid thrill is a difficult sign to be sure about. I have not found it helpful myself in the past in picking up ascites. What is the most specific diagnostic sign of fluid in the abdomen?
Student	I don't know.
Consultant	Ballotement or 'dipping', when you can feel your fingers dipping through the fluid onto the liver. This is an excellent sign often present when there is a lot of fluid, but, regrettably, I have found over the years that this sign is frequently neglected by students — and, I might add, by housemen too! Would you like to try it in Mrs C.?

The student tries 'dipping' into Mrs C.'s abdomen and is delighted when he finds the sign is positive.

Consultant	Any other abnormality in the abdomen?
Student	I found it difficult to be sure about any of the other abdominal organs because of the ascites.
Consultant	I appreciate the difficulty. What particular organ would you be interested in?
Student	The kidneys would obviously be relevant if we think that Mrs C. has renal failure.
Consultant	What renal abnormality might you find on palpation in a patient with renal failure?
Student	The kidneys could be enlarged in polycystic disease.
Consultant	Yes, polycystic disease is certainly a cause of renal failure in the third and fourth decades. Do you know the two other common presentations of polycystic disease?
Student	Haematuria is one of them but I can't remember the other one.
Consultant	The other one is hypertension. However, as far as I am aware, polycystic disease of the kidneys never presents as a nephrotic syndrome. Now, let us get back to your examination findings and perhaps you might tell us about Mrs C.'s heart and remember we are interested mainly in the question of heart failure.
Student	Her pulse was normal, BP 150/85, the apex beat was normal and I thought the heart sounds were normal with no murmurs.
Consultant	What about the jugular venous pressure which is an important indication of right ventricular failure?
Student	The neck veins were not distended and I thought that the jugular venous pressure was therefore normal.
Consultant	The absence of a raised jugular venous pressure makes right ventricular failure very unlikely. You found Mrs C.'s blood pressure was normal. Does the normal blood pressure tell us anything about the question of renal disease?
Student	The blood pressure is usually raised in renal disease.
Consultant	Hypertension is almost always associated with chronic renal disease so that Mrs C.'s normal blood pressure would indicate that any renal disease she might have is unlikely to have been present for many years. Now what about her lungs?
Student	I thought they were normal.
Consultant	What changes might you expect in the lungs in right ventricular failure?
Student	You would expect to find extensive basal crepitations.
Consultant	No, I think you are confusing right ventricular failure with left ventricular failure when you do get basal crepitations due to pulmonary congestion. Of course, long-standing left ventricular failure can eventually lead to right ventricular failure so you might hear basal crepita-

tions in these circumstances. To return to my original question what signs might you find in the lungs in right ventricular failure?

Student   I'm not clear what you mean.

Consultant   In Barnsley particularly, but also in many other areas in the North, right ventricular failure is frequently due to chronic obstructive airway disease, so what I was wanting you to say was that there was no evidence of chronic bronchitis or emphysema which might lead to right ventricular failure, or as it is more commonly known in chronic lung disease, cor pulmonale.

Finally, what about the nervous system — did you find any evidence of a uraemic peripheral neuropathy?

Student   There was no muscle weakness and all the reflexes were normal.

Consultant   What about the sensory system?

Student   I didn't test for this.

Consultant   That's a shame because the peripheral neuropathy of renal failure is usually a sensory type and not motor; some experts think it leads to the so-called 'restless legs syndrome'. The other interesting thing about uraemic polyneuropathy is that it occurs more frequently in patients on chronic haemodialysis. Anyway Mrs C. does not have any evidence of sensory neuropathy.

At this point I think that we can summarize our conclusions from the examination findings:

EXAMINATION

- we have confirmed marked pitting oedema of the legs
- the puffiness round Mrs C.'s eyes suggest a renal origin for her oedema (nephrotic syndrome)
- she has evidence of ascites which would support the possibility of nephrotic syndrome
- there is no evidence of right ventricular failure to account for the oedema
- Mrs C. looks anaemic and this might be due to renal failure associated with the nephrotic syndrome

---

Consultant   Now I would like to consider the investigations necessary to elucidate Mrs C.'s diagnosis. What are your views on this?

Student   I think we should start with a blood count and ESR.

Consultant   That is always the first test suggested by students for any case.
In what way will the blood count and ESR help?

Student   We have said that she is likely to be anaemic and the blood count should give us some help here.

Consultant   The haemoglobin is likely to be useful but I doubt whether the white

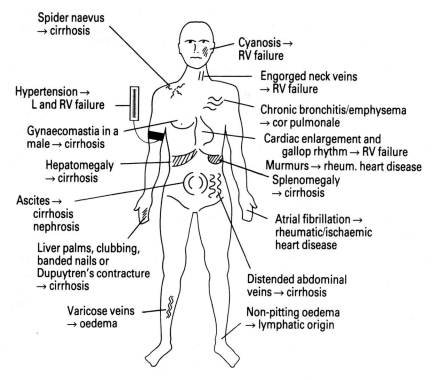

Figure 4.1 Possible signs of diagnostic help in a patient with oedema.

count will help. A raised ESR may show an acute inflammatory state or neoplasia, but is really so non-specific as to be of very limited help.

Here is the result of Mrs C.'s blood count; I want you to tell me what you think.

		Normal range
Haemoglobin	11.2	11.5–16.5 g/dl
White cell count	8500	$4.0–11.0 \times 10^9/mm^3$
ESR	12	7–15 in 1 hr

Student	The blood count confirms mild anaemia though from the figures you have given me it's not possible to say what type. The white count and the ESR are normal.
Consultant	The blood count has not really helped very much in diagnosing Mrs C.'s problem, has it?
	What would be a more useful test if you suspect that a patient has oedema which may be of renal origin?
Student	You want to know whether she has any albumin in the urine.

Consultant	Exactly. So the first test is a simple urine examination 'to see if she has heavy albuminuria which would indicate nephrotic syndrome. When I was a student we were expected to do our own regular urine examinations — all the wards had a small testing room attached where students and housemen could do these simple tests. I regret the passing of this commendable practice — it taught us all self-reliance.
Student	I have looked at the laboratory urine test result and this does confirm that Mrs C. has heavy albuminuria.
Consultant	What urinary loss of albumin is required over 24 hours before nephrotic syndrome develops?
Student	I think it's about 3 grams.
Consultant	Not quite right, 3.5 grams in 24 hours is the minimum loss required to produce hypo-albuminaemia and therefore oedema. What other proteins might be lost in the urine in nephrotic syndrome and does it matter anyway?
Student	I don't know. I've never been asked that question before.
Consultant	In a severe case of nephrotic syndrome, you can get loss of *thyroxine-binding globulin* though thyroid function remains unchanged, *transferrin* leading to iron-deficiency anaemia, *antithrombin III* leading to venous thrombosis and *cholecalciferol-binding protein* leading to bone disease. What blood test should we do to confirm nephrotic syndrome?
Student	We should measure the level of serum albumin.
Consultant	Right. Mrs C.'s serum albumin on admission was 22 g/L. Is this normal?
Student	No, it is low — it should be at least 35 g/L.
Consultant	So this confirms the diagnosis of nephrotic syndrome. Should we do any more tests?
Student	I think we should carry out an IVP.
Consultant	How will this help?
Student	It will confirm nephrotic syndrome because you can get enlargement of the kidneys.
Consultant	This may sometimes be seen in nephrotic syndrome but again it is too non-specific to be of any real value. A more important aspect of the IVP in Mrs C. would be to show whether renal function is satisfactory and adequate dye is excreted. However, we could be a bit more accurate in assessing Mrs C.'s renal function by doing another test, couldn't we?
Student	By measuring the blood urea.
Consultant	That is a rather crude index of renal function; the more sensitive measurement would be ...
Student	The serum creatinine level.
Consultant	That's right. An even better test would be to measure the creatinine

clearance but this may overestimate the glomerular filtration rate in nephrotic syndrome. Here are Mrs C.'s results:

		Normal range (mmol/L)
Blood urea	9.9	3.3–6.6
Serum creatinine	149	60–100

What do you think of these results?

Student

Both the blood urea and the creatinine levels are increased, indicating that Mrs C. does have renal failure.

Consultant

The renal failure is relatively mild and would be unlikely to lead to anaemia. Are there any other blood tests which may be abnormal in nephrotic syndrome?

Student

The cholesterol level may be increased.

Consultant

Mrs C.'s total cholesterol was 9.6 mmol/L (normal 3.6–6.7) and the triglyceride level was 3.5 mmol/L (normal 0.6–1.7) so this confirms your view that her blood lipids are raised and is further supporting evidence that she has nephrotic syndrome.

Now, where do we go from here in the way of tests?

Student

All the evidence so far suggests nephrotic syndrome and the only way to prove it would be by renal biopsy.

Consultant

I agree. A renal biopsy would be the most useful test of all — it will confirm the diagnosis, though I don't think this is in doubt, but more importantly it will show us the type and degree of histological damage which will influence treatment and prognosis.

Have you any idea what the renal biopsy might show in nephrotic syndrome?

Student

All I could remember of the histology is that you can get a membranous type of glomerular nephritis.

Consultant

Good, that's probably one of the commonest histological types of nephrotic syndrome — *a membrano-proliferative change* in the glomerulus. There are three other likely pathological types — the *minimal lesion of lipoid nephrosis, the membranous type which is not proliferative*, and the most serious type of all, *the focal proliferative type* which can be either a *segmental type of glomerular sclerosis* or a rapidly *progressive glomerular nephritis*.

Mrs C.'s renal biopsy showed focal segmental glomerular sclerosis.

Do you know the causes of nephrotic syndrome?

Student

It can occur in diabetes and, I think, in collagen diseases like systemic lupus erythematosus.

Consultant

Do you know any other name for nephrotic syndrome associated with diabetes?

Student	Intercapillary glomerulosclerosis.
Consultant	That's very good but I had another name in mind.
Student	I'm sorry I don't know.
Consultant	It's called the Kimmelstiel–Wilson* syndrome. Are there any other causes of nephrotic syndrome?
Student	It can be due to primary renal disease.
Consultant	In fact, in over 80% of cases of nephrotic syndrome there is so-called idiopathic glomerular lesions, which means that we are not sure of the cause though it seems likely that the basis of the lesion is an auto-immune reaction in the glomerulus; what the trigger is remains unclear.
	There are other specific causes in the remaining 20%. You have mentioned diabetes and collagen disease: other causes include drugs (like gold, penicillamine, captopril), amyloidosis, sarcoidosis, renal vein thrombosis and neoplasia (like Hodgkin's[†] disease, carcinomatosis and leukaemia).
	As far as Mrs C. is concerned, we think she fits into the idiopathic auto-immune type of nephrotic syndrome.
	Now if we can turn to the consideration of treatment. What are your recommendations?
Student	Well, firstly, I think she should have diuretics to get rid of the oedema.
Consultant	It might be better to divide the treatment into symptomatic and specific treatment. Diuretics come under symptomatic treatment. If you do use diuretics on Mrs C. is there any special hazard to watch out for?
Student	One of the important side-effects might be hypokalaemia.
Consultant	That would apply particularly with a loop diuretic such as frusemide or bumetanide. On the other hand, if she is given spironolactone the important thing to watch for is hyperkalaemia, especially if there is associated renal failure. Another side-effect of diuretics in nephrotic syndrome is, paradoxically, oliguria and an increase in renal failure, especially with the loop diuretics.
	Is there any other symptomatic treatment which might be helpful in Mrs C.?
Student	She should restrict her salt intake.
Consultant	Do you have any figure in mind?
Student	I'm really not sure.
Consultant	Do you know what the average daily intake of salt is in the UK?

* P. Kimmelstiel (1900–1970) was an American pathologist; C. Wilson is a contemporary English physician, born in 1906, who worked at the London Hospital, though he is now retired.
† Thomas Hodgkin (1798–1866) was a pathologist at Guy's Hospital. He studied with Laennec in Paris and was the first to introduce a stethoscope to Guy's Hospital. R.T.H. Laennec (1781–1826) was a French physician whose major claim to fame is that he invented the stethoscope.

Student	I think it's about 10 grams a day.
Consultant	That's right. Mrs C. should reduce this at the very least to no more than 3 g daily, which means cutting out all added salt at the table, though it is still allowed in the cooking. If her oedema is very resistant to treatment she may have to reduce this even further to under 1 gram a day and this will mean excluding salt altogether from the cooking — the food won't taste very nice I can assure you! Any other symptomatic treatment?
Student	I can't think of any.
Consultant	Well, in an emergency, you could give her some intravenous albumin. It would be indicated especially if she had a reduced circulating blood volume in the presence of significant hypotension. It is only of temporary value since the infused albumin is soon lost from the circulation. Now what about specific treatment for the renal lesion and I'm referring particularly to Mrs C.'s kidney lesion which you will remember is likely to be of the auto-immune type?
Student	You could give her steroids.
Consultant	Steroids are most likely to be of value if the glomerular lesion is minimal, but unfortunately minimal change disease, though very common in children, occurs in only 20% of adults. The dose of prednisolone used to treat nephrotic syndrome, whether in children or in adults is 1 mg/kg/day. Other drugs are also sometimes used in treatment — do you know which?
Student	I'm sorry I don't.
Consultant	Cyclophosphamide is sometimes used in prednisolone-resistant cases but you have to watch out for bone marrow suppression. Azathioprine is an alternative to cyclophosphamide but its main action is in reducing the requirements for large doses of prednisolone.

OUTCOME

Mrs C. was started on prednisolone 20 mg tds together with frusemide 40 mg bd. There was initial improvement in her oedema, a reduction in abdominal girth due to lessening of the ascites and a fall in body weight.

Unfortunately, the proteinuria persisted although it reduced to 1.0–1.5 g/L. The prednisolone was continued for one month in steadily reducing doses and then discontinued since there was no further reduction in the albuminuria.

Over the next 12 months the oedema remained under reasonable control with the frusemide, but the blood urea steadily increased and she was referred to a nephrologist for consideration of renal transplantation.

LEARNING POINTS

Commonest causes of bilateral leg oedema

- heart failure
- nephrotic syndrome
- cirrhosis

Symptoms of renal failure

- polyuria/nocturia
- excessive thirst
- nausea and vomiting
- diarrhoea
- hiccups
- twitching
- bleeding tendency
- drowsiness/confusion/coma

Causes of polyuria

- renal failure
- diabetes mellitus
- diabetes insipidus
- hyperparathyroidism
- psychogenic

Anaemia in renal failure

- reduced erythropoiesis
  lack of erythropoietic factor
  uraemic bone marrow depression
- gastro-intestinal bleeding from uraemic colitis
- impaired platelet function → bleeding
- deficiency of iron and folate in the diet
- increased haemolysis due to abnormal plasma factor

Signs of ascites

- abdominal distension in the flanks
- everted umbilicus
- shifting dullness
- fluid thrill
- ballottement (dipping)

Clinical presentation of polycystic disease of the kidneys

- hypertension
- haematuria
- uraemia

Relevant investigations in nephrotic syndrome

- urine examination for albuminuria
- serum albumin level (<3.5 g/L)
- blood urea/serum creatinine for renal failure
- blood lipids for hyperlipidaemia
- IVP for renal function
- renal biopsy for glomerular histopathology

Urinary loss of protein in nephrotic syndrome

- albumin → oedema
- thyroxine-binding globulin (thyroid function normal)
- transferrin → iron-deficiency anaemia
- antithrombin III → venous thrombosis
- cholecalciferol-binding protein → bone disease

Causes of nephrotic syndrome

- infection
  streptococcal
  syphilis
  hepatitis B
- drugs
  gold
  penicillamine
  tridione
  captopril
- systemic disease
  diabetes mellitus
  collagen disease
  sarcoidosis
  amyloidosis
  Henoch–Schönlein* purpura
- malignancy
  Hodgkin's[†] disease
  leukaemia
  carcinomatosis
- renal vein thrombosis

Glomerular histopathology in nephrotic syndrome

- minimal lesion
- membranous

* E.H. Henoch (1820–1910) was a German paediatrician; J.L. Schönlein (1793–1864) was a German physician, a contemporary of Virchow.
† Thomas Hodgkin (1798–1866) was a lecturer in pathology at Guy's Hospital.

- membrano-proliferative
- focal proliferative — segmental
  progressive glomerulonephritis

Treatment of nephrotic syndrome

- symptomatic
  diuretics
  salt restriction
  albumin infusion
- specific
  prednisolone
  cyclophosphamide
  azathioprine

Guidelines in assessing response to treatment in nephrotic syndrome

- fall in body weight
- lessening of oedema
- reduction in urinary protein excretion
- increase in serum albumin concentration
- fall in serum creatinine concentration

5

Indigestion

Student	Mrs A.B. is a 63-year-old lady who has been admitted for investigation of indigestion.
	She has suffered with indigestion on and off for over 20 years since she had a gastric ulcer diagnosed on a barium meal when she was about 40 years old. The indigestion has been giving her very little trouble over the last few years until it became severe again. She is complaining of pain in the upper part of the abdomen which is sometimes related to eating and at other times occurs quite independently of meals. It has awakened her at night and sometimes she has vomited when the pain has been particularly bad. She also said that she has occasionally seen streaks of blood in the vomit. She has tried indigestion mixtures like Aludrox but is not sure whether they help much. She has been off her food recently and thinks she has lost some weight as a result, though she is not sure how much. I asked about her bowels — she admits a bit of constipation recently but has not noticed any diarrhoea at any time.
	In the past history, she had some gallbladder trouble about 5 years ago — gallstones she thinks — and was advised to have her gallbladder out but she was afraid of having an operation and so she refused. She brings up a lot of wind and has rumbling in her abdomen which she says is relieved by drinking hot water. Her other big problem is arthritis which affects her hands and knees mainly; this has been troubling her for the last year or two and she has been taking indomethacin as well as aspirin to control the pain. She has also suffered with her neck for many years and sometimes has to wear a collar for this.
	There was nothing else of significance in the past history or in the family history. Mrs B. doesn't smoke and only drinks on special occasions.
Consultant	You have provided a lot of 'meaty' symptoms to get our teeth into — I hope you will forgive the rather poor pun.
	What are your thoughts on the history?
Student	The first thing that occurred to me was whether she had an exacerbation of her gastric ulcer.
Consultant	Yes, I think that is the first diagnosis to consider as we know that she

	had a gastric ulcer in the past, though we mustn't forget her gallstones. Did you think that the pain she described suggested ulcer-type pain?
Student	She said that it was a burning pain and it seems to me to be mainly in the epigastric area. I think that this could be ulcer pain.
Consultant	Yes, it could be, although typically ulcer pain is described as dull gnawing pain. What about the relationship to meals?
Student	It is not always related to eating.
Consultant	And do you think that this lack of consistent relationship to meals would exclude an ulcer?
Student	I am not sure. We were always taught that ulcer pain is related to meals — after meals for gastric ulcer and before meals for duodenal ulcer.
Consultant	I was taught the same. Experience, however, has taught me otherwise; ulcer pain can occur and often does occur without any relationship to eating at all. That's the trouble with traditional teaching sometimes — it fails to get modified in the textbooks in the light of practical experience. You mention quite rightly the difference between the timing of pain due to gastric ulcer and duodenal ulcer. Are there any other symptoms which could help to distinguish the two?
Student	The pain in duodenal ulcer is relieved by eating while gastric ulcer pain gets worse.
Consultant	Good. Anything else?
Student	Duodenal pain occurs at night, as in Mrs B.'s case.
Consultant	Do you know why?
Student	It's to do with high acid levels at night in patients with duodenal ulcer.
Consultant	That's correct. Duodenal ulcer is associated more frequently with increased gastric acidity than gastric ulcer, and this is particularly marked at night when the stomach is empty. Any other distinguishing points?
Student	Is vomiting more frequent in duodenal ulcer?
Consultant	No, it's the other way round unless the duodenal ulcer has produced stenosis of the pylorus. Can you think of any other clues to differentiate gastric and duodenal ulcer?
Student	No, I can't think of anything else.
Consultant	Another point worth mentioning is that pain in the back is much more common in duodenal ulcer than in gastric ulcer: it's due to erosion of the duodenal ulcer through to the pancreas. There is one other very important distinction between the two types of ulcer — a gastric ulcer can become neoplastic, while for all practical purposes, it never occurs with a duodenal ulcer. What about other possible diagnoses?
Student	I wondered whether she could have a recurrence of her gallbladder trouble.

Consultant	What type of abdominal symptom would you get in gallbladder disease?
Student	She seems to have chronic flatulent dyspepsia which is caused typically by chronic gallbladder disease.
Consultant	There I must take issue with you. It is a widespread fallacy that chronic gallbladder disease leads to so-called 'flatulent dyspepsia' — wind, abdominal distension, rumbling, nausea, etc. It has been clearly shown that not only are these symptoms as common in patients without gallbladder disease as those with, but also when cholecystectomy is carried out in those patients with these symptoms and gallbladder disease, it has little effect on the persistence or otherwise of the symptoms. No, the only time you get authentic abdominal pain due to gallbladder disease is when the patient has . . .?
Student	Gallstones.
Consultant	That's right — you get so-called 'biliary colic'. Why do I say 'so-called'?
Student	I don't know.
Consultant	Because the pain with gallstones is usually a constant and not a colicky pain. There is one other occasion when you get authentic gallbladder pain.
Student	In acute cholecystitis.
Consultant	Good. Can you tell us any distinguishing characteristics about gall-bladder pain?
Student	It usually occurs in the right hypochondrium.
Consultant	That is usually the site but it can also involve the epigastrium. What about the radiation of the pain?
Student	It can radiate to the tip of the right shoulder.
Consultant	Why is that?
Student	I think it's because it's referred pain through the phrenic nerve.
Consultant	Good. It is also often referred to the lower part of the right scapula. Is Mrs B.'s pain anything like true gallbladder pain?
Student	No, I don't think so.
Consultant	What other diagnoses should be considered?
Student	I wondered about an irritable bowel syndrome because of the complaint of a lot of wind and stomach rumbling.
Consultant	I agree that these symptoms are suggestive of an irritable bowel, but in my experience it is rare to get epigastric pain. Where is the usual site of the pain in irritable bowel syndrome?
Student	It usually affects the left iliac fossa.
Consultant	That is the commonest site of the pain. Other common sites include the left hypochondrium and the right iliac fossa. Are there any other diagnoses that we ought to consider in Mrs B.?

Student	There is always the possibility that she may have a neoplasm.
Consultant	I would agree, especially at this age; you will remember that we mentioned the possibility of such change occurring in a gastric ulcer. Are there any other symptoms to support this possibility?
Student	She said that she had lost weight.
Consultant	This could be significant, though when a patient with indigestion loses weight you must try to find out whether this is because the patient is afraid to eat while the appetite remains normal — such as often happens with a benign gastric ulcer — or whether it's because the appetite has been lost, such as occurs with neoplasia. Which do you think it is in Mrs B.'s case?
Student	I didn't actually ask her whether she was afraid to eat because of pain, but she did say that her appetite had been poor.
Consultant	This would support the possibility of a gastric neoplasm. Let me go off on a slightly different tack now. Is there anything else in the past history which might be relevant to her indigestion?
Student	I can't think of anything else at the moment.
Consultant	Let me put it another way: is there any possibility of iatrogenic disease?
Student	I'm not too sure what that means.
Consultant	Surely all medical students know the meaning of the Greek word *iatros*, from which the word iatrogenic is derived.
Student	I'm sorry, I never learned any Greek.
Consultant	I'll let you into a secret — neither did I; nor did I learn any Latin which all educated doctors did in days gone by. I'm pulling your leg really. *Iatros* is the Greek word for doctor and iatrogenic therefore means produced by the doctor. To return to Mrs B., is there anything that the doctor has given to her which might cause indigestion?
Student	Oh, I see what you mean now. She has been taking aspirin and indomethacin for her arthritis and these drugs lead to peptic ulcer.
Consultant	That's right, and we will have to keep this possibility in mind if we decide that her problem is due to a simple gastric ulcer. Is there another common cause of indigestion which we have not mentioned so far?
Student	Do you mean alcohol?
Consultant	No, I was not thinking of that, though alcohol can cause gastritis and indigestion. In any case it does not apply to Mrs B. because you told us she drinks little. What I'm thinking of occurs most frequently in obese patients and may be related to posture.
Student	You mean hiatus hernia.
Consultant	I do indeed. It's a very common cause of indigestion, or perhaps it would be more accurate to say 'heartburn'. Is Mrs B.'s indigestion related in any way to posture?

Student	I forgot to ask her — I'll ask her now. Mrs B., is your pain worse when you are bending down or lying down?
Consultant	Not the best way of asking the question — you have asked a leading question which wouldn't be allowed in a court of law. It would be better to ask her whether the pain is better or worse when she bends or lies down, so at least she has the choice of answer.
Student	Mrs B., does stooping or bending down make any difference to your pain?
Patient	No, I can't say that I have noticed any effect on the pain.
Consultant	It is unlikely therefore that Mrs B.'s pain is due to gastro-oesophageal regurgitation. Do you know any other condition which can cause epigastric pain — a condition unrelated to the stomach or oesophagus?
Student	Acute pancreatitis can cause severe epigastric pain.
Consultant	It can, but it doesn't go on for months on end.
Student	What about chronic pancreatitis?
Consultant	That's more like it. Do you know any distinguishing features about pancreatic pain?
Student	It can penetrate through to the back.
Consultant	That's correct. It resembles the pain produced by a penetrating posterior wall duodenal ulcer — in fact, it is pancreatic pain which is produced by ulceration through into the pancreas. Do you know any other diagnostic clue to pancreatic pain?
Student	I can't think of anything else.
Consultant	Pancreatic pain is worse lying down and better when the patient sits up. What other symptoms are associated with pancreatitis?
Student	You might get diarrhoea.
Consultant	And what is the cause of the diarrhoea?
Student	It's due to malabsorption.
Consultant	That's right. As well as causing diarrhoea the malabsorption can lead to deficiencies resulting in anaemia (iron, folic acid), bleeding (vitamin K), sore mouth (vitamin B), tetany (calcium) and osteomalacia (vitamin D). Mrs B. has none of these deficiencies. What is the usual cause of chronic pancreatitis?
Student	It can be due to chronic gallbladder disease.
Consultant	Any other factor?
Student	Alcoholism, I think.
Consultant	Yes, alcoholism and chronic gallbladder disease are the two main aetiological factors in this country. There is one other condition which occurs in children — I am sure you know what it is.
Student	Fibrocystic disease.

Consultant	That's right. Fibrocystic disease is a congenital condition and unfortunately many affected children will die young. However, some may survive long enough to show features of chronic pancreatitis. Now there is one other abdominal condition which is often overlooked and may also cause severe abdominal pain related to meals. I will give you a hint by saying that it occurs particularly in patients who are severely arteriosclerotic.
Student	Unfortunately the hint hasn't really helped me. I don't know what you have in mind.
Consultant	I'm thinking of superior mesenteric ischaemia. Do you know anything about this condition?
Student	I have heard of it but have never come across it. I suppose that it's due to insufficient blood supply to the bowel because of arteriosclerosis of the superior mesenteric artery.
Consultant	Yes, that is the cause. It is an uncommon condition but I have seen several cases. Do you know any of the symptoms?
Student	Well, obviously there is abdominal pain because you mentioned it but I don't know any other symptoms.
Consultant	Typically, it produces colicky central abdominal pain about 15 to 30 minutes after meals. There is one other important symptom which often occurs with the pain and helps the diagnosis — diarrhoea. Since Mrs B.'s pain is epigastric and not peri-umbilical, also she has no diarrhoea, I think we can exclude this diagnosis. The time has come for us to summarize our conclusions from the history and then we can go on with your examination findings:

HISTORY

- Mrs B. has a 20-year history of indigestion
- a gastric ulcer has been found previously
- she may have an acute exacerbation of her gastric ulcer
- her recent anorexia and loss of weight raises the possibility of neoplasia — either neoplastic change in a chronic gastric ulcer or occurring *de novo*
- she has symptoms of irritable bowel syndrome
- she has been taking aspirin and indomethacin for long-standing arthritis and this may also be a contributory factor in the indigestion
- there is a past history of gallbladder disease but this is not considered to be the cause of her present problems

Consultant	Now, I would like you to tell us your findings and do try to keep the likely diagnoses in mind when you do (Figure 5.1).
Student	She looks as if she has lost some weight and I thought she was anaemic. She doesn't look jaundiced. Her pulse was 84 and regular, the blood pressure was 150/100 . . .

Consultant	Could I stop you for a moment. Are the cardiovascular findings related to the indigestion?
Student	Not really, I suppse.
Consultant	Then can I remind you of the need to present your findings in a problem-orientated way; in the case of Mrs B. this means related to her gastro-intestinal system.
Student	All right I will go on to the abdominal findings then. She had definite epigastric tenderness and I thought I felt a vague mass in the upper abdomen, though I couldn't decide whether it was an epigastric mass or possibly the liver.

The consultant palpates the abdomen.

Consultant	I agree there is some difficulty in feeling her abdomen adequately because she relaxes poorly. It sometimes helps relaxation to ask the patient to bend the knees up and breathe through the mouth. I think myself that what you are feeling is more likely to be the left lobe of the liver about two fingers below the costal margin; it is quite firm and smooth. Carry on with your findings.
Student	I couldn't feel the spleen or kidneys.
Consultant	The kidneys are not really relevant to Mrs B.'s problems — you are slipping back into your routine presentation — try to keep problem-orientated. Any other findings?
Student	Not really.
Consultant	If Mrs B. had a neoplastic lesion in the stomach, are there any other signs which may occur?
Student	We have already mentioned the enlarged liver.
Consultant	We have. What else?
Student	She could have some enlarged glands.
Consultant	Which glands in particular?
Student	I think you can get enlargement of the left supraclavicular glands with a gastric neoplasm. I did feel her neck but couldn't feel any glands.
Consultant	Do you know what this particular gland is called and what the sign is called?
Student	I'm afraid not.
Consultant	The gland is called Virchow's gland and the sign is called Troisier's sign. I don't suppose I dare ask you who these medical gentlemen were.
Student	I'm sorry, I don't know.
Consultant	Rudolf Karl Virchow was a very famous German pathologist who lived 1821–1902 and wrote an important treatise on cellular pathology. Charles Émile Troisier was a distinguished French physician in Paris

and lived from 1844 to 1919; as well as the sign in the neck he is known for one of the earliest descriptions of haemochromatosis, also known as . . . ?

Student	I don't know any other name for haemochromatosis.
Consultant	Bronzed diabetes.

Now, I would like to turn to the other possible diagnoses which we discussed. You will remember that we considered gallbladder disease, hiatus hernia, chronic pancreatitis and mesenteric ischaemia.

What about her gallbladder?

Student	I couldn't feel her gallbladder.
Consultant	Would you expect to?
Student	You could if it was diseased.
Consultant	Do you mean if it was diseased due to chronic cholecystitis?
Student	Yes, I suppose so.
Consultant	Do you remember Courvoisier's* law?
Student	If you have a patient with obstructive jaundice and you can feel an enlarged gallbladder, then the obstruction can't be due to chronic cholecystitis.
Consultant	Do you know why this is so?
Student	Because the gallbladder becomes fibrosed and shrunken in chronic cholecystitis.
Consultant	That's right, and that is why you can't usually feel a chronically inflamed gallbladder. I suppose we ought to mention the one exception to Courvoisier's law — if there is an associated stone impacted in the common bile duct the gallbladder can sometimes swell up because of the development of a mucocoele.

To get back to Mrs B.'s gallbladder, if it was enlarged might you think of another pathology?

Student	It could be neoplastic.
Consultant	That's right. Were there any signs of the other diagnosis we mentioned, chronic pancreatitis?
Student	She is anaemic.
Consultant	This could be due to a gastric problem, benign or otherwise. You have to be more specific if you are thinking of signs of deficiency due to malabsorption in chronic pancreatitis. What about vitamin B deficiency?
Student	She hasn't got a sore mouth or sore tongue.

---

* J. Courvoisier (1843–1918) was Professor of Surgery in Basle and pioneered the surgery of the biliary tract — he was one of the first surgeons to remove a stone from the common bile duct.

Consultant	Good, but don't forget the other important clinical manifestation of vitamin B deficiency in the nervous system.
Student	You mean peripheral neuritis — she didn't have any abnormal neurological signs.
Consultant	What about calcium deficiency?
Student	I didn't think of testing for tetany.
Consultant	I think we agree that there is really no evidence of chronic pancreatitis, particularly as she doesn't have diarrhoea. Now, what about the other interesting diagnosis we have mentioned — superior mesenteric ischaemia. Were there any signs of this?
Student	I don't really know what signs you would look for.
Consultant	There are no diagnostic signs for mesenteric ischaemia; perhaps the closest we would come to it is by hearing a systolic murmur over the abdominal aorta which would indicate significant arteriosclerosis in the abdomen. You would of course also be likely to find signs of arteriosclerosis in the other peripheral vessels such as the radial, brachial, fundal and pedal arteries.
Student	I did check all her peripheral arteries and thought they were normal. I didn't think of listening over the abdominal aorta but I will remember it for next time.
Consultant	Is there anything else you want to tell us about in your examination?
Student	The heart and lungs were normal, and as I mentioned earlier I couldn't find any abnormality in her nervous system.
Consultant	How thoroughly did you check the nervous system?
Student	I checked her pupils, reflexes and plantar responses.
Consultant	Not exactly a thorough neurological examination! I will, however, let you get away with it this time but I would advise you strongly to do a detailed neurological examination if there is likely to be any neurological abnormality in the patient. We've now reached the stage of summarizing our findings:

EXAMINATION

- Mrs B. has epigastric tenderness which could suggest an active gastric ulcer or oesophagitis
- there may be liver enlargement which would suggest the possibility of neoplasia
- there was no murmur over the abdominal aorta to indicate mesenteric ischaemia
- there were no signs of malabsorption which might be due to chronic pancreatitis
- she did not have Troisier's sign to suggest a gastric neoplasm

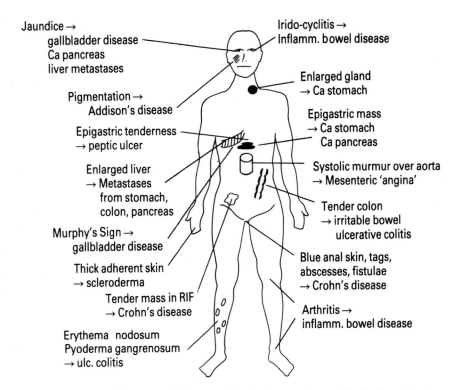

Jaundice →
  gallbladder disease
  Ca pancreas
  liver metastases

Pigmentation →
  Addison's disease

Epigastric tenderness
  → peptic ulcer

Enlarged liver
  → Metastases
  from stomach,
  colon, pancreas

Murphy's Sign →
  gallbladder disease

Thick adherent skin
  → scleroderma

Tender mass in RIF
  → Crohn's disease

Erythema nodosum
Pyoderma gangrenosum
  → ulc. colitis

Irido-cyclitis →
  Inflamm. bowel disease

Enlarged gland
  → Ca stomach

Epigastric mass
  → Ca stomach
  Ca pancreas

Systolic murmur over aorta
  → Mesenteric 'angina'

Tender colon
  → irritable bowel
  ulcerative colitis

Blue anal skin, tags,
abscesses, fistulae
  → Crohn's disease

Arthritis →
  inflamm. bowel disease

Figure 5.1   Possible signs of diagnostic help in a patient with 'indigestion'.

Consultant	I think that we should now turn our attention to the question of investigation. What would you suggest we do first?
Student	I think we should start with a full blood count.
Consultant	What would you be looking for?
Student	For anaemia.
Consultant	I think that's reasonable; you did mention that she was pale and a gastric lesion of whatever type can certainly cause anaemia. Mrs B.'s haemoglobin was 9.9 g/dl; what does this tell you?
Student	It confirms that she is anaemic.
Consultant	What kind of anaemia?
Student	You can't say without some more information.
Consultant	Try to be specific — what other blood results do you want?
Student	The blood film might help in showing the size of the red cells.
Consultant	The mean corpuscular volume would be a better indicator. The blood film is reported as microcytic, hypochromic anaemia.

Student	This indicates an iron-deficiency anaemia and could be due to bleeding from the alimentary tract.
Consultant	I agree. What other tests would you like?
Student	An ESR might be useful; if it was very high it might suggest a malignant lesion of the stomach, provided it is not due to an acute exacerbation of her arthritis.
Consultant	That is another good suggestion. Any other tests?
Student	What about liver function tests?
Consultant	They may help to show abnormal function but there are more relevant tests available. Have you any suggestions?
Student	An ultrasound test would show liver enlargement.
Consultant	It would and it might also show whether there were any deposits, so it is well worth doing. Mrs B.'s test did in fact confirm hepatomegaly but did not suggest any focal lesion which might be due to a metastatic deposit.
	Now, the tests we have discussed so far have given us some useful information, but we have not yet mentioned the most important test of all in Mrs B. What would that be?
Student	A barium meal examination.
Consultant	A barium examination might give us an answer but there is an even better test available for Mrs B. — which?
Student	You mean gastroscopy?
Consultant	That's right. Gastroscopy would be a better test because if Mrs B. had a gastric lesion, which is what we expect, then not only will gastroscopy be able to show us the lesion but also give us an opportunity to biopsy it.
	We have done both tests in Mrs B. First I will show you the barium meal and invite your comments (Figure 5.2).
Student	There seems to be a filling defect on the greater curve of the stomach.
Consultant	What do you think it is?
Student	I would think that the most likely diagnosis is a gastric neoplasm.
Consultant	Yes, that would certainly be the first condition to consider. Does the fact that it is on the greater curve of the stomach tell you anything about its origin?
Student	I'm not sure what you are getting at.
Consultant	If the lesion was on the lesser curve of the stomach rather than the greater curve it might suggest that there could have been a predisposing condition.
Student	I think I know what you mean now. A neoplasm on the lesser curve could be the result of neoplastic change in a pre-existing gastric ulcer.
Consultant	Yes, that's what I have in mind. A greater curve lesion of this kind is more likely to be neoplastic *de novo*; if it occurs on the lesser curve then

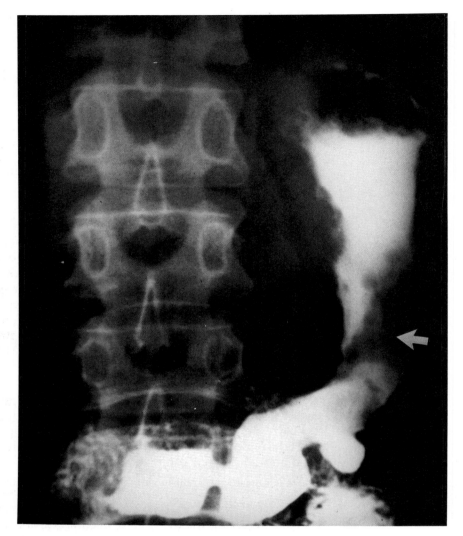

Figure 5.2 Barium meal showing a large filling defect on the greater curve of the stomach due to a carcinoma (arrowed).

the chances are that it has developed as a result of neoplastic change in a chronic gastric ulcer. On this basis, Mrs B. is likely to have a new lesion and not one arising in her old gastric ulcer.

Now, before I tell you the result of Mrs B.'s gastroscopy perhaps we ought to mention briefly what other investigations are required for the other diagnoses that we discussed in the differential diagnosis. First of all, gallbladder disease.

Student   I think that a cholecystogram would probably be the best test.

Consultant	I wouldn't consider it the first test to do; what about a straight X-ray of the abdomen — would that help? (Figure 5.3).
Student	It might show gallstones.
Consultant	It might indeed. Do you know how often you are likely to see radio-opaque gallstones?
Student	In about 50% of cases, I believe.
Consultant	You are a bit optimistic — more like 30%. It is with renal stones that you get a higher percentage of stones visible on a straight abdominal X-ray, 70%. If you don't see stones on the X-ray, then what would be your next test?
Student	A cholecystogram?
Consultant	Possibly — I would prefer an ultrasound test. Do you know what for?
Student	It could show any gallstones.
Consultant	Yes, it can show stones as small as 3 mm. It may also show intra-hepatic dilatation of the bile ducts that indicates obstruction and often implies a surgically-remediable cause. The other tests for gallbladder disease include, as you mentioned, cholecystography, intravenous cholangiography if the gallbladder is non-functioning or has been removed, and, one of the most recent techniques, endoscopic retrograde cholangiopancreatography (ERCP) which also allows removal of the stones as well in some circumstances. What about diagnosing hiatus hernia?
Student	A barium meal or gastroscopy will show a hiatus hernia.
Consultant	To correct you slightly, a barium meal may show a hernia but gastroscopy is mainly of use in showing the accompanying oesophagitis. What tests would you use to diagnose pancreatic disease?
Student	Malabsorption tests are probably best.
Consultant	Yes, tests for fat content of the stools and the xylose excretion test are useful in diagnosing chronic pancreatitis. If you suspect a neoplasm, then a barium meal may help by showing distortion of the duodenal loop, and abdominal ultrasound or a radio-active scan of the pancreas may also be useful. One other simple test worth keeping in mind is once again the humble straight X-ray of the abdomen which may show pancreatic calcification indicating chronic pancreatitis. Superior mesenteric ischaemia is a difficult diagnosis to confirm — how would you do it?
Student	I suppose by arteriography.
Consultant	Good. It requires selective catheterization of the superior mesenteric artery.

In view of the malignant nature of Mrs B.'s problem the consultant considers it better to retire to ward-sister's office for further discussion.

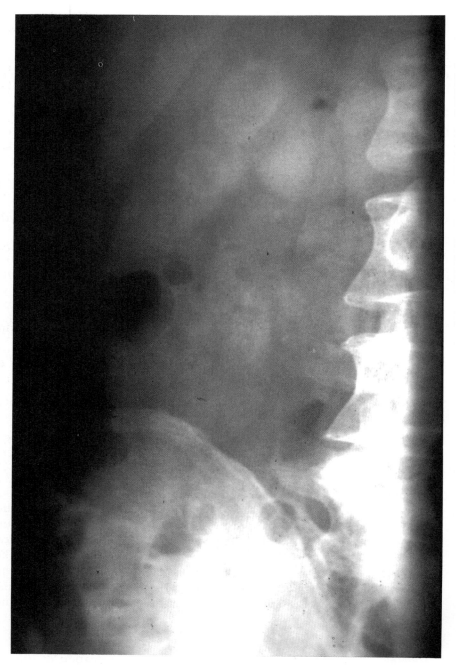

Figure 5.3 Straight X-ray of the abdomen showing gallstones.

Consultant	Now, I think we should return to Mrs B.'s problem. Gastroscopy with biopsy has confirmed the diagnosis. What are your thoughts on treatment?
Student	I think that the best form of treatment would be an operation.
Consultant	I would agree though experience shows that radical surgery is very rarely feasible. Certainly if there is any doubt about the diagnosis or about possibility of resection, then, at the very least, there should be an exploratory laparotomy. Usually, however, by the time the patient has presented with symptoms the neoplasm has spread extensively and operation is not feasible. Perhaps we ought just to finish off still on a surgical note by considering what the indications are for surgery in a benign gastric ulcer.
Student	The first indication would be if repeated medical treatment failed to control symptoms and heal the ulcer.
Consultant	That is obviously an important indication and probably one of the most frequent reasons for surgery. What other indications?
Student	If there are any complications of the ulcer.
Consultant	What complications do you have in mind?
Student	Well, obviously if there was a perforation or bleeding that couldn't be controlled with medical treatment.
Consultant	Good, and also don't forget obstruction as a result of the ulcer, especially pyloric stenosis. There is one other important indication which is exemplified by Mrs B.
Student	If you suspect that the ulcer may be malignant.
Consultant	That's right, though usually you should be able to make this decision better on the result of a biopsy taken at gastroscopy. The final point I want to emphasize is the importance always of ensuring that a gastric ulcer has healed satisfactorily following any medical treatment you have given, and this means an objective assessment of healing by gastroscopy. Do you know why I am making this point?
Student	Because there is always the possibility of the gastric ulcer being malignant.
Consultant	And on that final correct answer I think we can stop.

OUTCOME

In the absence of any clinical evidence of metastases, it was decided to carry out a laparotomy to see whether operative treatment was feasible.

Unfortunately at laparotomy it was obvious that the gastric carcinoma had spread to involve the adjacent lymph nodes, and it was also thought likely that there were two small metastatic deposits in the liver.

No operative treatment was possible and Mrs B. deteriorated rapidly after the laparotomy and died in 6 weeks.

LEARNING POINTS

Differentiation between gastric and duodenal ulcer

	Gastric ulcer	*Duodenal ulcer*
Relation to meals	1–2 hr after	just before
Effect of eating	pain worse	pain better
Night pain	rare	common
Penetration through to the back	rare	sometimes
Appetite	poor (afraid to eat)	normal
Vomiting	common	rare (unless pyloric stenosis occurs)
Weight loss	may occur due to fear of eating	rare

Barium meal compared with gastroscopy in the diagnosis of peptic ulcer

	Barium meal	*Gastroscopy*
Advantages	simple inexpensive widely available	accurate distinguishes between benign and malignant ulcers can take biopsy can assess healing can control bleeding (diathermy)
Disadvantages	misses ulcer (20–30%) poor differentiation between benign and malignant ulcers biopsy not possible	not readily available uncomfortable complications occur — oesophageal perforation perforation of ulcer restart bleeding ulcer

Clinical features of superior mesenteric ischaemia

- periumbilical colicky pain
- occurs 15–30 minutes after meals
- associated with diarrhoea

Indications for gastroscopy

- failure to respond to medical treatment
- equivocal barium meal

- to assess response to treatment
- to exclude malignancy
- to detect and possibly treat cause of bleeding
- to detect an ulcer when previous stomach operation makes barium meal unhelpful

Investigation of gallbladder disease

- straight X-ray of the abdomen — radio-opaque stones (30%)
- abdominal ultrasound for biliary dilatation or gallstones
- cholecystography — identifies 70% of stones
- intravenous cholangiography — especially if previous cholecys-tectomy
- ERCP — allows removal of some stones through sphincterotomy

Investigation of pancreatic disease

- straight X-ray abdomen — may show pancreatic calcification
- barium meal for deformity of duodenal loop
- tests of malabsorption
    fat
    iron
    calcium
    folate
    carbohydrate (xylose)
- abdominal ultrasound
- radio-isotope studies

Indications for surgery in peptic ulcer

- failed medical treatment
- suspicion of malignancy in gastric ulcer
- complications
    perforation
    uncontrolled bleeding
    pyloric stenosis
- unacceptable disruption of work/leisure

6

Diarrhoea

Student

Mr T.S. is a 42-year-old firearms instructor who has been admitted for investigation of a recent exacerbation of long-standing diarrhoea.

His diarrhoea started about 6 years ago and occurs in attacks lasting several weeks at a time; the bowels are normal between the attacks. During the bouts of diarrhoea, he has 3 to 4 motions a day, the stools are loose and he has noticed blood sometimes but thinks this could be due to piles which he has had for a long time. In the latest attack, for which he has been admitted this time, he says that the diarrhoea is a lot worse, up to 12 times a day, and he has noticed a lot more blood than usual. He also complains of colicky abdominal pain when he has diarrhoea; the pain is in the lower part of the abdomen though he sometimes feels it in the left or the right iliac fossa as well. He had a barium examination 2 years ago and he was told that the bowel was 'clear'.

His appetite is not very good at present and he thinks he has lost about a stone in weight over the past 3 months. He has not been vomiting and the rest of the systematic enquiry was negative.

In the past, he has had problems with his nerves which has been bad enough on two occasions for him to see a psychiatrist. He still takes regular diazepam. Otherwise, there have been no serious illnesses or operations.

In the family history, he has had two uncles who died of cancer of the bowel in their fifties, and he admits that he is very worried in case he has the same problem. He doesn't smoke and drinks moderately — about 5 or 6 pints of beer a week. As far as treatment is concerned, apart from the diazepam, he only has codeine tablets for the attacks of diarrhoea and these have been prescribed by his own doctor.

I think those are all the relevant facts I could find out in the history. Do you want me to go ahead with the examination findings?

Consultant

No, not at the moment. We should always try to make a diagnosis from the history in any medical problem and then use the examination to confirm the diagnosis, to add to the diagnosis or to refute the diagnosis suggested by the history. So I would like you to tell us what you views are, based on Mr S.'s symptoms.

Student

It could be infective.

Consultant	What type of infection do you have in mind that would go on for 6 years?
Student	It could be dysentery.
Consultant	What kind of dysentery?
Student	Bacillary dysentery.
Consultant	Bacillary dysentery, due to Shigella, is an acute condition in the great majority of cases and tends to occur where sanitation is poor; it rarely becomes chronic — some experts say never.
	Amoebic dysentery, on the other hand, does cause a subacute or chronic disorder and is usually picked up in hot countries where sanitation is poor — has Mr S. ever been in any countries of this kind?
Student	I'm afraid I didn't ask him.
Patient	No, I've only been abroad on holiday to Europe — I've never been to the Tropics.
Consultant	It is of course possible to get dysentery in some countries in Europe where sanitation is very poor.
	Are there any other infections that can lead to chronic diarrhoea?
Student	Tuberculosis of the bowel.
Consultant	Tuberculosis can affect the gastro-intestinal tract, usually in the ileo-caecal region. In the UK most patients with a tuberculous bowel will be Asian immigrants, or very elderly, so it's very unlikely in Mr S.'s case.
	Other possible infective causes of chronic diarrhoea include Yersinia, especially in Scandinavian countries, Campylobacter, which sometimes leads to bleeding into the bowel also, and *Giardia lamblia* infestation.
	Let's leave infective causes of chronic diarrhoea now because they are very rare in this country except in institutions. What are the other more likely possibilities in Mr S.?
Student	He could have a neoplasm in the bowel.
Consultant	I would agree that you should always think of a neoplasm in a patient with bloody diarrhoea and loss of weight. However, the length of history — 6 years — obviously makes this diagnosis untenable unless the neoplasm has developed recently as a complication of a more chronic underlying disease of the bowel.
	Now you mentioned that Mr S. had trouble with his nerves — could that have any bearing on his diarrhoea?
Student	Could he have irritable bowel syndrome?
Consultant	That's an interesting suggestion but not exactly what I had in mind. Irritable bowel syndrome, or spastic colon, does occur in anxious individuals and causes abdominal pain, diarrhoea or constipation or both, as well as nausea, abdominal distension and rumbling.
	In my experience, irritable bowel is much more frequent in women than men but that doesn't of course exclude it in Mr S. There is, however,

	a much more important part of Mr S.'s history which virtually excludes a spastic colon — what do you think that might be?
Student	You don't get blood in stools in spastic colon.
Consultant	That's right — bloody diarrhoea doesn't occur in irritable bowel syndrome, but you must remember that piles are common and often coexist with an irritable bowel and may therefore lead to some superficial blood on the surface of the stool. Incidentally, when you mention rectal bleeding as you did in your initial presentation, you should always try to distinguish between blood on the surface of the stool — which would suggest piles — and blood mixed in with the stool — which indicates the likelihood of disease of the bowel itself.
	The other important symptom in Mr S. which makes irritable bowel very unlikely is his loss of weight which is also not a feature of this condition.
	Let's have some more possible causes of chronic diarrhoea.
Student	He may be suffering from malabsorption syndrome.
Consultant	What particular symptom would make you suspect malabsorption in a patient?
Student	The nature of the stools — they would be bulky and offensive.
Consultant	And they would be very difficult to flush away. Does Mr S. have stools like that?
Student	No, I don't think so — he said that his motions were loose and watery though I didn't ask him specially about how they flushed away.
Consultant	It's an important question. Mr S., can you tell us the answer?
Patient	I haven't noticed any difficulty like that — the motions always seem to flush away without any difficulty.
Consultant	Thank you, Mr S. It appears very unlikely that Mr S. has malabsorption syndrome. Perhaps we should mention briefly the other symptoms which may be associated with malabsorption — can you think of any?
Student	You would get symptoms due to vitamin deficiency.
Consultant	What vitamins do you mean?
Student	I'm thinking of vitamin B, which can cause beri-beri, and also vitamin K, which can lead to bleeding.
Consultant	It is very unlikely that vitamin B deficiency would be severe enough to cause beri-beri; it would be much more likely to cause no more than a sore tongue and angular stomatitis.
	Vitamin K deficiency can certainly lead to bleeding as a result of inadequate synthesis of prothrombin.
	What other deficiencies can occur?
Student	Tetany can occur due to lack of absorption of calcium.
Consultant	That's right. What else?

Student	Iron-deficiency anaemia due to a lack of iron, or macrocytic anaemia caused by deficiency of folic acid.
Consultant	What other causes should we consider now for Mr S.'s diarrhoea?
Student	I think we ought to think of inflammatory bowel disease.
Consultant	And by this you mean ...?
Student	Ulcerative colitis or Crohn's* disease.
Consultant	What are the distinctive features of these conditions?
Student	Both conditions cause bloody diarrhoea associated with abdominal pain. You can also get severe constitutional disturbances like fever and loss of weight. There may also be complications in other systems away from the abdomen.
Consultant	That's not a bad résumé; the only point I would add about the bloody diarrhoea is that it is less marked in Crohn's disease than in ulcerative colitis. If we think that Mr S. might have inflammatory bowel disease, which of the two conditions do you think it is likely to be?
Student	The site of the abdominal pain might help.
Consultant	Would you like to amplify that answer?
Student	The pain in ulcerative colitis is usually on the left side of the abdomen over the descending colon while Crohn's disease causes pain in the right iliac fossa.
Consultant	That's right. Pain arising in the small bowel is usually felt around the umbilical area, while colonic pain occurs either in the lower part of the abdomen or either side of the abdomen depending on whether the ascending or descending colon is affected. In Mr S.'s case, you said he had both central abdominal pain and pain in either of the iliac fossae so which of the two inflammatory bowel conditions do you think more likely?
Student	The site of the pain would suggest involvement of both the small bowel and the large bowel — this is more likely to occur in Crohn's disease than in ulcerative colitis which only affects the colon.
Consultant	I would agree that Mr S.'s abdominal pain is more suggestive of Crohn's disease than ulcerative colitis. The anorexia and weight loss also support this diagnosis, since these symptoms are a lot more common than in ulcerative colitis. Do you think there might be any more relevant symptoms worth enquiring about specifically from Mr S. to help us decide whether he could have inflammatory bowel disease?

* B.B. Crohn (1884–1983) was an American gastroenterologist who described his new disease in 1932. He worked at the Mount Sinai Hospital in New York.

Student	Yes, we could ask whether he has any symptoms of the complications associated with ulcerative colitis and Crohn's disease.
Consultant	Like what?
Student	He could have pain in his joints.
Consultant	Yes, arthritis can occur in about 20% of patients; it tends to affect only one joint at a time, often the knee. Does any other type of arthritis occur, especially in Crohn's disease?
Student	Yes, you can get ankylosing spondylitis.
Consultant	That's right. It often starts out with pain over the sacro-iliac joints due to sacro-iliitis. Does Mr S. have any pain in his joints or his spine?
Student	I'm sorry, I didn't think to ask him. Mr S., can you tell us whether you have had any back pain or pain in any other joints?
Patient	As a matter of fact I have been having a bit of pain recently in the bottom of my back, especially when I bend — I thought I was getting rheumatism.
Consultant	We will have to check up further on this back pain — it could be relevant. Perhaps you might give us some more information when you present your examination findings. Do you know any other systemic complications of inflammatory bowel disease?
Student	You can get rashes in the skin.
Consultant	Could you be more specific?
Student	Erythema nodosum can occur.
Consultant	This occurs in both ulcerative colitis and Crohn's disease. Unlike ankylosing spondylitis, erythema nodosum is related to the activity of the disease at the time. Do you know any other skin complications?
Student	Pyoderma gangrenosum.
Consultant	That is always mentioned in the books and every student seems to remember it. In fact I have never seen it although I have dealt with a large number of patients with ulcerative colitis, so I think it must be very rare. Can you think of any other complications?
Student	Not apart from local complications like perforation and haemorrhage.
Consultant	There are several other systemic complications of inflammatory bowel disease, like painful eyes due to conjunctivitis, episcleritis or uveitis, and also liver involvement leading to sclerosing cholangitis, pericholangitis, chronic active hepatitis, cirrhosis and gallstones. Can we get back now to other causes of chronic diarrhoea? You said in your history that Mr S. has colicky central abdominal pain with the

	diarrhoea. Is there any other condition you can think of which can cause this type of pain accompanied by diarrhoea? Let me give you a clue: the pain and the diarrhoea in this condition occur about 20 to 30 minutes after eating.
Student	I don't suppose you mean a gastric ulcer?
Consultant	No, that doesn't cause either peri-umbilical pain or diarrhoea. If I told you further that it occurs particularly in elderly arteriosclerotic individuals, would that help?
Student	I'm sorry I'm still not sure what condition you have in mind.
Consultant	I'm referring to superior mesenteric ischaemia, and the condition is sometimes also called 'mesenteric angina'; it's often forgotten in the differential diagnosis of chronic diarrhoea.
	Are there any drugs which may cause chronic diarrhoea?
Student	Excessive use of laxatives would be the first drugs I would think of.
Consultant	What else?
Student	Antibiotics cause diarrhoea.
Consultant	Although that is usually short-term diarrhoea, sometimes *Clostridium difficile* pseudo-membranous colitis can go on for prolonged periods leading to a more chronic diarrhoea.
	What other causes of chronic diarrhoea? Let me try to help you again — what about drugs for high blood pressure?
Student	Methyldopa can sometimes cause diarrhoea.
Consultant	It can but, in my experience, it doesn't happen very often.
	Any other blood pressure drugs causing diarrhoea?
Student	I'm sorry I don't know.
Consultant	Beta-blockers, especially atenolol, can occasionally lead to diarrhoea, but again in my experience, this is uncommon.
	Can you think of any other drugs in common use, apart from antihypertensives, which can cause diarrhoea?
Student	Digoxin.
Consultant	Yes, that's an important one, especially in elderly patients.
	Any others?
Student	I can't think of any at the moment.
Consultant	Non-steroidal anti-inflammatory drugs are often forgotten as a cause of diarrhoea — you should always keep them in mind particularly when you remember the large number of patients on this therapy.
	Tell me some other causes of chronic diarrhoea — endocrinological ones for example.
Student	Thyrotoxicosis.
Consultant	Another good textbook cause but very rare in practice in my experience. Did you ask Mr S. if he has any symptoms of thyrotoxicosis?

Student	No, because I didn't think of this diagnosis.
Consultant	We won't bother asking him as I don't think that this diagnosis is at all likely, but I would like you to remind us briefly of the relevant symptoms.
Student	The patient would complain of heat intolerance, excessive sweating, tremors and loss of weight. He might also notice protrusion of his eyes.
Consultant	Very good. Can you think of any other endocrine cause of chronic diarrhoea?
Student	I can't think of any other cause.
Consultant	Diabetes is another important cause — do you know under what conditions?
Student	Is it a symptom of diabetic neuropathy?
Consultant	Good. It is due to autonomic neuropathy occurring in diabetes. An interesting fact about this type of diarrhoea is that it tends to be worse at night. Do you know any other important symptom of diabetic autonomic neuropathy, which might help in diagnosing the condition?
Student	I'm sorry I don't.
Consultant	Postural hypotension with dizziness is the symptom I have in mind. Has Mr S. any symptoms to suggest that he may be a diabetic?
Student	I don't think so. He has no polyuria though I didn't ask him about polydipsia. Mr S., have you noticed that you are more thirsty than normal and drinking more fluids?
Patient	I can't say that I have.
Consultant	Bearing in mind the symptom we were just talking about — postural hypotension — is there any other condition which comes to mind to consider as a cause of chronic diarrhoea? Remember we are still thinking endocrinologically!
Student	I'm sorry, no.
Consultant	If I told you the patient might have a colour problem, would that be of any help?
Student	I'm still not clear what condition you mean.
Consultant	I'm referring to Addison's* disease, the main features of which are pigmentation, extreme fatigue, postural hypotension and gastrointestinal symptoms like diarrhoea. Do you think that Mr S. could be suffering from Addison's disease?
Student	He isn't pigmented and he wasn't complaining of excessive fatigue when I was taking his history.

---

* Thomas Addison (1793–1860) was a physician at Guy's Hospital and described his adrenal disease in 1855.

| Consultant | Perhaps you might comment further on this diagnosis in your examination. |

Other rarer endocrinological causes of chronic diarrhoea include carcinoid syndrome and various gastrointestinal tumours associated with the release of vasoactive polypeptides, e.g. insulinoma, gastrinoma, glucagonoma (these are often designated VIPomas).

To complete the list of causes of chronic diarrhoea, we should mention the bacterial overgrowth in the bowel, especially in old people with chronic bowel stasis, and we mustn't forget amyloid disease, which occurs with chronic rheumatoid arthritis and chronic suppurative conditions. I think we have considered the main causes of chronic diarrhoea so perhaps we could try to summarize our conclusions:

HISTORY

- Mr S. has chronic, episodic diarrhoea with a recent severe exacerbation
- chronic infection from amoebiasis or tuberculosis is considered very unlikely though Yersinia and Campylobacter cannot be ruled out on the history alone
- the long history rules out neoplastic disease of the bowel except possibly as a recent complication of pre-existing disease
- the nature of the stools does not suggest malabsorption
- there is nothing to suggest diabetic neuropathy, thyrotoxicosis or drugs as a likely cause
- inflammatory bowel disease remains the most likely diagnosis, and the distribution of the abdominal pain suggests Crohn's disease rather than ulcerative colitis
- possible support for this diagnosis is the recent development of low backache which might be due to ankylosing spondylitis and/or sacro-iliitis

---

| Consultant | Now I would like you to tell us your examination findings and I want you to concentrate on the diagnosis we thought most likely on the basis of the symptoms, which you will remember was inflammatory bowel disease (Figure 6.1). |

| Student | Mr S. is pyrexial with a temperature of 38.8°. The conjunctivae look pale, suggesting anaemia. I couldn't find any enlarged glands in the neck or axillae. His pulse is 96 and regular, blood pressure 135/75. The apex beat was normal, the heart sounds were normal with no murmurs, the lungs were clear ... |

| Consultant | Forgive me for interrupting you. |

You quite rightly started your examination with general observations on anaemia and pyrexia which are obviously relevant in a patient with possible inflammatory bowel disease. However, I was not so happy about your subsequent routine presentation going through the systems, as so many students seem taught to do. I think it better to go on to the examination of the system likely to be involved, as suggested by the history; in Mr S.'s case, his abdomen, not forgetting of course the other extra-abdominal complications of inflammatory bowel disease. You can tell us about the other systems later, and I appreciate that the cardiovascular system may be important in assessing fluid loss and hypovolaemia.

Try to present a problem-orientated examination whenever you can.

Student	The abdomen was generally soft and there was tenderness in both iliac fossae. I thought that he had a vague swelling in the right iliac fossa, but I wasn't too sure and I didn't want to press too hard because he was tender at this spot. I could also feel the descending colon, which was definitely tender. I couldn't feel either the liver or the spleen.
Consultant	How do you explain these findings?
Student	The tender descending colon would be in favour of ulcerative colitis.
Consultant	That's true but don't forget that you may also get involvement of the colon in Crohn's disease. Also you found tenderness in the right iliac fossa — what does that suggest?
Student	This would be more in favour of Crohn's disease.
Consultant	I agree. What about the lump in the right iliac fossa?
Student	That is also in favour of Crohn's disease, but I did say that I wasn't too sure of this.
Consultant	In fact you are right — he does have a mass in the right iliac fossa which all of us have felt; this is strongly suggestive of Crohn's disease which you will remember starts usually in the terminal ileum. Before we leave the lump in the right iliac fossa, don't forget the other possibilities such as a neoplasm in the caecum, and more rarely, a carcinoid mass. Did you do a rectal examination?
Student	I tried but Mr S. said it was very painful so I didn't persist.
Consultant	You have done well to try. It is an important part of the examination in inflammatory bowel disease. Mr S., do you mind if we have a look at your back passage; we won't try an internal examination so we won't be hurting you. What can you see?
Student	He has a few anal tags.
Consultant	That might be relevant since this is a feature which tends to occur in Crohn's disease. Do you notice anything else about the anal region?
Student	He doesn't have any abscesses or fistulae.
Consultant	That's a good observation, since both of these complications can occur in Crohn's disease. What do you think about the colour of the peri-anal skin?

Student	It looks a bit blue.

Consultant	That is also a sign which occurs commonly in Crohn's disease — bluish induration in the peri-anal region.
	    Thank you Mr S., please turn round on your back again.
	    Now, having considered the most relevant part of the examination in Mr S., the abdominal findings, can you give some thought to the possible complications of Crohn's which we discussed earlier?

Student	He hasn't any evidence of arthritis.
Consultant	Did you test his spine or sacro-iliac joints?
Student	No, I didn't think he was fit to get out of bed.
Consultant	You got out of that one very nicely! You could of course test the sacro-iliac joints in bed, though I agree not the spine. What about his eyes?
Student	They seem alright — there was no local redness or tenderness.
Consultant	And the skin?
Student	He doesn't have erythema nodosum or pyoderma gangrenosum.
Consultant	Here's one we didn't mention before — what about his mouth?
Patient	I have been getting a lot of ulcers in my mouth lately.
Consultant	Mr S., you've given the game away! (To student) Did you have a look inside his mouth?
Student	Yes, but I didn't see any ulcers.
Consultant	Did you look for them?
Student	No, I must own up that I didn't look specifically for ulcers in the mouth.
Consultant	Mouth ulcers do occur in Crohn's disease but are very rare in ulcerative colitis. The history of mouth ulcers gives us more support for the diagnosis of Crohn's disease. There is one other sign that is worth mentioning — you would find it in the hands.
Student	He doesn't have any finger clubbing.
Consultant	Good. Finger clubbing occurs both in Crohn's disease and ulcerative colitis but as you know it is a non-specific sign and can occur in a variety of other diseases of cardiac, pulmonary and gastrointestinal origin — would you care to name some of them?
Student	Clubbing occurs in bronchial neoplasm and other chronic lung disease like tuberculosis and bronchiectasis.
Consultant	Don't forget lung abscess as well. Go on.
Student	You can get it in congenital heart disease and also in subacute bacterial endocarditis.
Consultant	It is congenital *cyanotic* heart disease. You're doing well — carry on.

Student	We have already mentioned inflammatory bowel disease and I think it can also occur in cirrhosis.
Consultant	Especially biliary cirrhosis. The other gastrointestinal condition in which you may get clubbing is idiopathic steatorrhoea. Finally, we should mention familial clubbing which is rare. To return to the examination findings, were the other systems all normal — you have already told us about the cardiovascular system so what about the respiratory and nervous systems?
Student	I couldn't find any abnormality in either.
Consultant	There is one other sign you mentioned — that Mr S. was anaemic. What do you think is the cause?
Student	It could be due to bleeding in the bowel.
Consultant	Yes, that is the most likely cause. Can you think of any other possible cause?
Student	No, I'm sorry.
Consultant	Crohn's disease can lead to malabsorption of folic acid which can result in a macrocytic anaemia. Of course, you can also get impaired absorption of vitamin B_{12} which is normally absorbed in the terminal ileum, but this would take a long time to cause a macrocytic anaemia wouldn't it?
Student	I'm not sure.
Consultant	Vitamin B_{12} is stored in the liver and there is usually at least a two-year supply, so it would take at least this time for the patient to become deficient and develop anaemia. The other factor contributing to anaemia is the chronic inflammatory disease itself. Well, I think that we are now in a position to summarize the important findings and the conclusions that we have drawn from them:

EXAMINATION

- Mr S. has tenderness in the right iliac fossa associated with a mass which is strongly suggestive of Crohn's disease
- he has a bluish discoloration in the perianal region and anal tags which supports this diagnosis
- the tenderness over the descending colon would suggest that the large bowel is likely to be affected also
- although the spine was not examined, there was no evidence of any systemic complications of Crohn's disease affecting the peripheral joints, skin, eyes or liver
- Mr S. is pale and is likely to be anaemic either as a result of gastrointestinal blood loss or due to folic acid deficiency

---

Consultant	Now, how should we set about confirming Mr S.'s diagnosis by investigation?

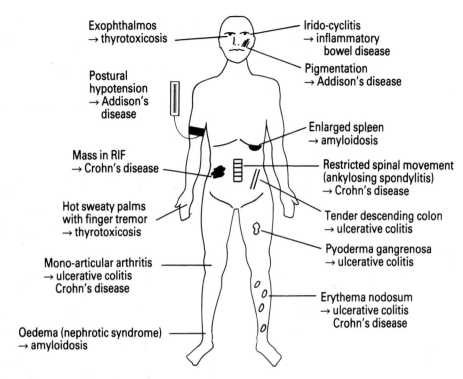

Exophthalmos
→ thyrotoxicosis

Irido-cyclitis
→ inflammatory
bowel disease

Pigmentation
→ Addison's disease

Postural
hypotension
→ Addison's
disease

Enlarged spleen
→ amyloidosis

Mass in RIF
→ Crohn's disease

Restricted spinal movement
(ankylosing spondylitis)
→ Crohn's disease

Hot sweaty palms
with finger tremor
→ thyrotoxicosis

Tender descending colon
→ ulcerative colitis

Pyoderma gangrenosa
→ ulcerative colitis

Mono-articular arthritis
→ ulcerative colitis
Crohn's disease

Erythema nodosum
→ ulcerative colitis
Crohn's disease

Oedema (nephrotic syndrome)
→ amyloidosis

Figure 6.1 Possible signs of diagnostic help in chronic diarrhoea.

Student	An X-ray examination of the bowel would help.
Consultant	It may indeed, but before we start calling on others to help the diagnosis is there anything that we might be able to do to help ourselves?
Student	We could carry out a sigmoidoscopy.
Consultant	That is what I had in mind. What do you think we might see?
Student	The mucosa might be inflamed and ulcerated.
Consultant	That's right, but these findings apply if Mr S. had ulcerative colitis, since all you are likely to see in Crohn's disease is mild hyperaemia or possibly no changes at all.

The changes seen in ulcerative colitis on sigmoidoscopy depend on the severity of the condition: in the mildest form all you will see is a hyperaemic and oedematous mucosa, and this will progress to a red granular mucosa with contact bleeding, and finally the changes you mentioned with actual ulceration.

Apart from the visual help we get from sigmoidoscopy, is there any other diagnostic value in this test?

Student	Yes, you would also do a biopsy of the rectal mucosa.

Consultant	Good. This is an important test and is the best way of trying to differentiate between ulcerative colitis and Crohn's disease which is often a difficult task. Do you know any of the distinguishing biopsy features between the two conditions?
Student	The ulcers in ulcerative colitis are superficial and in Crohn's disease they are deep.
Consultant	That is correct. Any other changes?
Student	That's all I can remember at the moment.
Consultant	Well, as you point out colitic ulcers are confined to the mucosa, whereas the ulcers in Crohn's disease are often transmural: the mucosal glands are commonly involved in ulcerative colitis producing crypt abscesses whereas this is much less frequent in Crohn's disease and finally you can see granulomata with giant cells in Crohn's disease but not in ulcerative colitis. Now, I would like to return to the question of X-ray examination of the bowel; what in particular do you want to X-ray?
Student	I think we should start with a barium enema.
Consultant	It would be better to do a straight X-ray of the abdomen first; in ulcerative colitis you may see the ragged, oedematous ulcerated mucosa in an air-filled colon, and in Crohn's disease you may see fistulae, so you could get useful diagnostic help from this simple investigation. What is the next test to do?
Student	I think we should then do the barium enema.
Consultant	I would agree. What changes would you expect to see in ulcerative colitis?
Student	You can sometimes see the ulcers in the descending colon.
Consultant	That is so and I have a barium enema film for you to see which shows this very well (Figure 6.2). Any other changes in the barium enema in ulcerative colitis?
Student	I'm not sure.
Consultant	Well, here is another X-ray which shows another typical sign — the bowel involvement by the ulcerative colitis is continuous and the haustrations are lost causing a long tube-like appearance in the colon (Figure 6.3). What about the changes in the barium enema in Crohn's disease?
Student	I can remember something about 'cobblestones'.
Consultant	Yes, that is an important feature when the large bowel is involved in Crohn's disease; it may be applicable to Mr S. since we suspect that his colon is affected. It is due to the deep transverse linear ulcers which occur in the colon separating off areas of the mucosa and giving the appearance of 'cobblestones'.

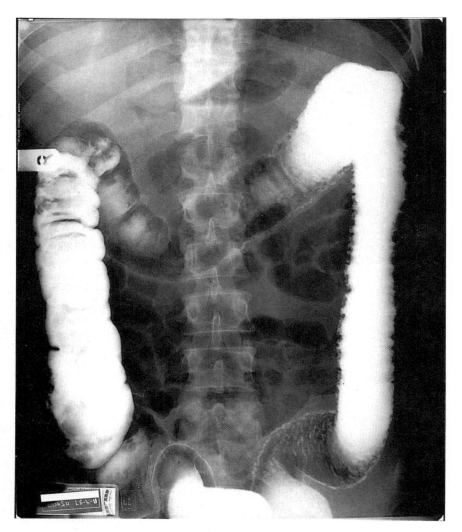

Figure 6.2 Barium enema in acute ulcerative colitis showing 'shagginess' of the mucosa in the descending colon due to acute ulceration.

	There are other radiological features in the colon in Crohn's disease — do you know any of them?
Student	I know that you can get strictures and fistulae.
Consultant	Good, and the other very suggestive sign is 'skip' lesions due to segmental involvement so that some areas of the mucosa are normal and lie adjacent to diseased areas.
	Is there any other radiological investigation which will help in the diagnosis of Crohn's disease?

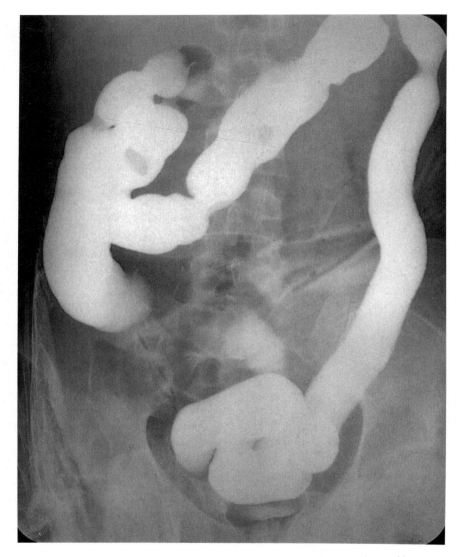

Figure 6.3 Barium enema in chronic ulcerative colitis showing loss of haustration in the descending colon giving the appearance of a straight-sided tube.

Student   The best test is likely to be a barium meal and follow-through examination.

Consultant   Ideally, you should have what is called a small bowel enema when the patient swallows a tube which ends up in the small bowel and the contrast material is then put down the tube — it produces a better picture of the small bowel than the usual follow-through examination. Unfortunately, not all X-ray departments use the tube technique.

It is the ileum which is predominantly affected in Crohn's disease; the changes are similar to those in the large bowel with 'skip' lesions, 'cobblestones' deep transverse fissures, strictures, dilatations and sometimes fistulae.

Here are Mr S.'s small bowel X-rays which show involvement of the terminal ileum and also of the colon which is what we suspected on clinical grounds (Figure 6.4).

Are there any other X-rays which might be useful in Mr S.?

Student	We could X-ray his spine for evidence of ankylosing spondylitis.
Consultant	Don't forget also to include an X-ray of the sacro-iliac joints for sacro-iliitis. Let's leave X-rays now and perhaps you can tell us about any other tests which you think might be helpful in the diagnosis of inflammatory bowel disease.
Student	I would think that a blood count and ESR could help.
Consultant	In what way?
Student	Mr S. is anaemic so it would confirm that and perhaps also indicate the type of anaemia.
Consultant	Yes, I agree that would be useful. What about the ESR?
Student	This would tell us how active the condition is.
Consultant	What about the white cell count?
Student	That would also give an indication of the activity of the disease.
Consultant	I think that the white count would be too non-specific to be of any real value; in any case the ESR would be a more reliable indication of disease activity. Do you want any other tests?
Student	I can't think of any more.
Consultant	Colonoscopy might be helpful, especially if you are in doubt about the differentiation between ulcerative colitis and Crohn's disease, as it may show ulcers especially in Crohn's disease and it enables biopsies to be taken from multiple sites in the colon. Tell me about the complications of Crohn's disease.
Student	We have already mentioned strictures and fistulae.
Consultant	Yes, those are the commonest complications. Strictures can lead on to dilatation, as in Mr S.'s X-rays, or more seriously, to actual intestinal obstruction. What effect might the disease have on absorption?
Student	It can cause malabsorption.
Consultant	Malabsorption is a well-known complication of Crohn's disease. Another uncommon complication is involvement of the right ureter leading to renal problems. Do you ever get neoplastic change in Crohn's disease?

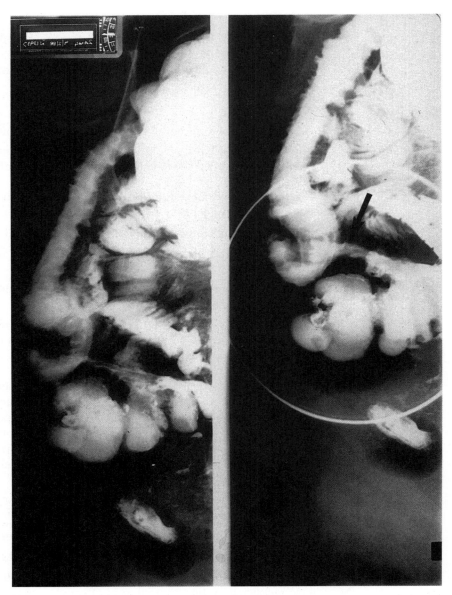

Figure 6.4 Small bowel enema in Crohn's disease showing a narrow constricted terminal ileum (arrowed).

Student	I don't know.
Consultant	Neoplasm of the small bowel is a very rare complication; you can get a neoplasm of the large bowel if the colon is affected, but obviously this is much rarer than in ulcerative colitis.

Now I wonder if we can turn our thoughts to the question of treating Mr S.'s Crohn's disease. How would you approach this?

Student	You can use steroids.
Consultant	Steroids are an important part of the treatment, but it might be more helpful if you separate the treatment for mild disease and a severe attack. How do you assess the severity of an attack of Crohn's disease?
Student	First of all by the severity of the diarrhoea.
Consultant	What else?
Student	As we mentioned earlier the ESR and the white count may help.
Consultant	The level of the haemoglobin would also give an indication of the severity of the disease. The degree of pyrexia is the other important guide to disease activity.
	Do you think that sigmoidoscopy might give us any useful information about the activity of the disease?
Student	It could do in ulcerative colitis but it is not so helpful in Crohn's disease.
Consultant	Do you think that the systemic complications give us any indication of disease activity?
Student	You said that erythema nodosum and the arthritis are related to the activity of the disease.
Consultant	That is correct, and the other complication that is similarly related is eye involvement. On the other hand, the complications which are unrelated to disease activity include ankylosing spondylitis, sacro-iliitis and the hepatic involvement.
	As far as the severity of Mr S.'s condition is concerned, he has a temperature of 38.8°, he looks ill, has lost weight, is anaemic and his bowels are open up to 12 times daily, so I think we shall regard him as having a severe attack. He doesn't have any skin or eye complications but he does have low back pain which might be due to early spinal involvement.
	Now to return to the question of treatment, what drugs do we have available to treat Crohn's disease?
Student	Apart from steroids which I mentioned earlier, we could also use sulphasalazine (Salazopyrin).
Consultant	And when would you use that in preference to steroids?
Student	I think you would use Salazopyrin if the attack was mild.
Consultant	It has been found of value in controlling exacerbations of Crohn's disease, especially when the colon is affected, but there is no convincing evidence that it prevents relapses.
	Do you know anything about how Salazopyrin works?
Student	Isn't it a combination of salicylic acid and a sulphonamide?
Consultant	That's right. The active therapeutic principle of sulphasalazine is 5-amino-salicylic acid (5-ASA), and it is combined with sulphapyridine, which acts mainly as a carrier to get the 5-ASA to the large bowel.
	5-ASA is available now on its own as mesalazine — the main indication for this preparation is in patients who are sensitive to sulphonamides and therefore are unable to take the combined preparation.

Other newer drugs have been developed for inflammatory bowel disease, like resin-coated 5-ASA and olsalazine, which may have advantages over sulphasalazine but they are not yet available in the UK.

The other drug worth mentioning is metronidazole, especially if there is perianal involvement in Crohn's disease or superadded bacterial infection. The disadvantage of metronidazole is the side-effects, including a reversible peripheral neuropathy, an antabuse-like reaction if the patient takes alcohol and gastrointestinal disturbances.

When would you use steroids?

Student   I suppose when you have a severe attack.

Consultant   Yes, in a severe attack you will need systemic steroids — you would usually start with intravenous hydrocortisone until the disease starts to come under control and then follow up with oral prednisolone for 6 to 8 weeks. You could also use local steroid enemas in a mild attack.

Do you know any other drugs which are sometimes used in Crohn's disease?

Student   I think you can use immunosuppressive drugs in some cases.

Consultant   That is true. Azathioprine is the immunosuppressive drug that is used but its main function is a 'steroid-sparing' one, to allow you to use a smaller dose of prednisolone and so reduce also the likelihood of side-effects: it has little therapeutic value on its own. If you do use azathioprine you must watch the blood count carefully for signs of bone-marrow suppression.

Before we leave the medical treatment of Crohn's disease to discuss the surgical approach, we mustn't forget the general treatment of the condition. Would you like to elaborate on this?

Student   You should treat any dehydration by intravenous fluids such as saline.

Consultant   That is important. It may be necessary to give another type of intravenous treatment if required — what is that?

Student   You might need to give him a blood transfusion if he is severely anaemic.

Consultant   Any other intravenous fluids necessary?

Student   I can't think of any.

Consultant   Total parenteral nutrition, or hyperalimentation as it is sometimes called, may be useful in really severe cases, especially if there is gross malnutrition.

The final aspect of treatment I would like you to consider is surgery for inflammatory bowel disease. What are your views on this, and we will extend this question to both ulcerative colitis and Crohn's disease?

Student   Surgery is required if the patient is completely resistant to all forms of medical treatment.

Consultant   I agree entirely with that indication; unfortunately the patient is often kept too long on medical treatment instead of considering surgery and the results may consequently be very poor.

	There are of course other very important indications for surgery in inflammatory bowel disease, aren't there?
Student	If there are any acute complications like perforation.
Consultant	That's right, also for intractable bleeding, both of which are more common in ulcerative colitis than in Crohn's disease.
	There is another very important complication in ulcerative colitis which requires urgent surgery — do you know what it is?
Student	Toxic megacolon.
Consultant	Well done! Are there any other local complications requiring surgery?
Student	If the patient develops a fistula.
Consultant	This occurs mainly in Crohn's disease — it is very rare in ulcerative colitis. Similarly, abscesses in Crohn's disease may require surgery if they don't settle satisfactorily with antibiotics.
	What about surgery for long-term complications of inflammatory bowel disease?
Student	You can get neoplastic change developing in ulcerative colitis.
Consultant	That's right. It occurs particularly in long-standing ulcerative colitis — at least 10 years' duration — and especially if the whole of the colon is involved (pancolitis). In fact, it is advisable to review regularly all patients with long-standing pancolitis for the development of neoplastic change; if any suspicious polyps are seen at colonoscopy or in a barium enema they should be removed.

The main long-term complication of Crohn's disease which may require surgery is stricture, especially if it is causing any intestinal obstruction.

The prognosis after surgery is more favourable in ulcerative colitis than in Crohn's disease.

We will finish at this point with a reminder I have learned, often to my cost, that the differential diagnosis of ulcerative colitis and Crohn's disease can be very dificult. You can never be 100% sure of the diagnosis even if all the clinical, radiological and even rectal biopsy features point to a particular diagnosis — the final arbiter is direct vision with detailed histology obtainable only at operation.

OUTCOME

Treatment was started with intravenous glucose-saline to correct dehydration and he was also given supplementary potassium to combat hypokalaemia. The degree of anaemia did not warrant a blood transfusion.

In view of the severity of the diarrhoea and a high ESR of 105 mm/hr he was treated initially with intravenous hydrocortisone 100 mg iv every 8 hours for 5 days, followed by 20 mg of prednisolone 8-hourly by mouth. On this régime he improved progressively, and the diarrhoea steadily reduced so that by the end of the first week of treatment bowel movements were down to 2 or 3 actions a day. His raised temperature settled within 48 hours and the ESR reduced to 35 mm/hr at the end of the first week and came down to normal in 2 weeks.

At the time of discharge he was feeling much better and his bowels were more or less normal; the dose of prednisolone had been reduced to 10 mg tds and it was decided to continue this dose until he was reviewed in the out-patient department in 2 weeks. At this review his improvement was maintained and he was started on Salazopyrin tablets 1.0 g four times daily, and he was advised to reduce the dose of prednisolone by 5 mg each day until he was off treatment in 6 days.

He was maintained successfully on a maintenance dose of Salazopyrin.

LEARNING POINTS

Causes of chronic diarrhoea

- infection
    amoebic dysentery
    tuberculosis of the bowel
    bacterial overgrowth in the elderly
    Yersinia
    Campylobacter
    Clostridium difficile
- irritable bowel syndrome
- malabsorption
- inflammatory bowel disease
- superior mesenteric artery ischaemia
- drugs
    non-steroidal anti-inflammatory agents
    magnesium-containing antacids
    digitalis preparations
    guanethidine (for hypertension)
    excessive purgatives
- endocrine
    thyrotoxicosis
    diabetes (autonomic neuropathy)
    Addison's disease
    carcinoid
    VIPomas

Clinical differentiation between ulcerative colitis and Crohn's disease

	Ulcerative colitis	*Crohn's disease*
Abdominal pain	lower abdomen	central abdomen
	left iliac fossa	right iliac fossa
Diarrhoea	severe	mild
Bleeding	profuse	mild
Abdominal mass	absent	frequent
Peri-anal disease	absent	frequent
Malabsorption	absent	sometimes
Mouth ulcers	rare	frequent
Back pain (ankylosing spondylitis)	rare	more likely

Systemic complications of inflammatory bowel disease

- skin lesions
    erythema nodosum
    pyoderma gangrenosum
- eyes

       conjunctivitis
       episcleritis
       uveitis

- arthritis
       mono-articular
       ankylosing spondylitis
       sacro-iliitis
- hepato-biliary
       sclerosing cholangitis
       pericholangitis
       chronic active hepatitis
       cirrhosis
       gallstones

Sigmoidoscopic changes in ulcerative colitis

- mild
       hyperaemia/oedema
- moderate
       red granular mucosa
       contact bleeding
- severe
       spontaneous bleeding
       mucosal ulceration

Histological differentiation between ulcerative colitis and Crohn's disease

Ulcerative colitis	*Crohn's disease*
Mucosal changes	transmural changes
Crypt abscesses common	crypt abscesses rare
—	granulomas
Polymorph infiltration	giant cell infiltration

Radiological comparison between ulcerative colitis and Crohn's disease

	Ulcerative colitis	*Crohn's disease*
Rectum	always involved	involved in 50%
Type of ulcer	shallow	deep linear
Extent of disease	continuous	segmental 'skip' lesions 'cobblestones'
Complications	acute — toxic megacolon	sinuses
	chronic — pseudo-polyps	strictures
	carcinoma	fistulae

Assessment of severity of inflammatory bowel disease

- frequency of diarrhoea
- degree of pyrexia
- amount of weight loss
- complications — arthritis
  erythema nodosum
  pyoderma gangrenosa
  eye involvement
- tests   — anaemia
  high ESR
  low serum albumin
- procto-sigmoidoscopy (ulcerative colitis)

Treatment of inflammatory bowel disease

mild attack
- sulphasalazine (Salazopyrin)
- metronidazole (Crohn's disease)
- steroid enemas
severe attack
- general — iv fluid for dehydration blood transfusion for severe anaemia parenteral nutrition
- specific — steroids iv initially; oral 6–8 weeks
- ?antibiotics (e.g. erythromycin)

Indications for surgery in inflammatory bowel disease

- severe attack not responding to full medical treatment
- acute complications
  toxic megacolon (ulcerative colitis)
  perforation
  intractable haemorrhage
- other complications
  Crohn's disease
    strictures
    abscesses
    fistulae
  ulcerative colitis
    pseudo-polyps
    carcinoma
- chronic unresponsive symptomatic disease
- ? pancolitis of at least 10 years' duration

7

Jaundice

Student
Mrs E.S. is a 48-year-old lady who presented with a 3-month history of jaundice. She thinks that her yellow colour varies from day to day but overall it has been getting worse. Since the jaundice has been bad she has been feeling generally unwell, is losing her appetite and also thinks she is losing weight. She said also that her skin has been itching over the last few weeks. I also asked her about the colour of her stools and her urine, and she said she thought that the stools were getting paler but she hadn't noticed anything special about her urine.

In the past she had an attack of jaundice about 5 years ago: it lasted about 6 weeks altogether, she was not admitted to hospital, nor did she have any special treatment at the time. Since then she has had a lot of what she calls 'flatulence'; by this she means a lot of wind, distension and rumbling in her abdomen, especially after she has eaten any fatty food. She also suffers from high blood pressure and has been taking tablets for about 8 years — she can't remember their name. Her nerves are bad at times and she needs to take tranquillizers — she is taking diazepam at present and has been taking this drug for about 2 years.

In the family history, she has a sister who suffers from rheumatoid arthritis, and I forgot to mention that Mrs S. also has been having pains in her hands and knees over the past few months — she puts it down to 'rheumatism', but she is wondering whether she might be getting rheumatoid arthritis like her sister.

She doesn't smoke and drinks very little — only on special occasions, and that's all I got from the history.

Consultant
That's an interesting, if somewhat brief, history. What are your thoughts on the diagnostic significance of her various symptoms?

Student
The main problem bringing her in was the jaundice.

Consultant
What type of jaundice do you think it is?

Student
It sounds like an obstructive type of jaundice because she said that her stools were pale.

Consultant
That's right, and the other symptom that suggests that the jaundice is obstructive is. . .?

Student
Oh yes, the itching.

Consultant	Right again. What's the mechanism of the itching?
Student	I think it's supposed to be due to the bile salts being deposited in the skin and acting as an irritant.
Consultant	That's correct. You said that she has pale stools — putty-coloured is the classical description — which indicates obstructive jaundice. Does the urine help in diagnosing obstructive jaundice?
Student	Yes it does. If there is complete obstruction there is no urobilinogen in the urine.
Consultant	That is quite right, but it does not in fact alter the colour of the urine as noticed by the patient. I haven't found that the colour of the urine, as noticed by the patient, has been of much diagnostic help in the cases of jaundice that I have had to deal with through the years — unlike changes in the colour of the stools. Now, before we go on with the clinical assessment it might be helpful if you were to remind us of the physiology of bilirubin. You could start by telling us where it comes from.
Student	Bilirubin comes from the breakdown of haemoglobin in the red cells. This occurs in the spleen, liver and bone marrow.
Consultant	Yes, bilirubin is the globin-free, iron-free fraction of haemoglobin; chemically, it is a porphyrin. Go on.
Student	The bilirubin circulates to the liver and is excreted in the bile to reach the intestine. It is converted to stercobilinogen in the bowel. Some of the stercobilinogen is reabsorbed from the bowel back into the circulation and re-excreted in the urine as urobilinogen. The rest of the stercobilinogen is excreted in the stools as stercobilin which is responsible for the colour of the stool.
Consultant	That is a very learned account of bilirubin metabolism.
Student	Thank you, I did after all get the class prize in physiology in my pre-clinical course.
Consultant	I see I shall have to be very careful with my physiology pronouncements when you're around! We can now see why obstructive jaundice is associated with pale stools — bilirubin is prevented from entering the bowel so no stercobilin is produced to colour the stool brown. Additionally, since no stercobilinogen is present in the bowel none can be reabsorbed to be re-excreted in the urine as urobilinogen. So the findings in *complete* obstructive jaundice are pale stools, bilirubin in the urine but no urobilinogen. In practice you rarely get cases of complete obstruction so you often see a trace of urobilinogen in the urine. What is the urine like in prehepatic jaundice e.g. haemolytic jaundice?
Student	In haemolytic jaundice you don't get any bilirubin in the urine.
Consultant	That's why it is called acholuric jaundice. Do you know why there is no bile in the urine?

Student	I think it is something to do with the conjugation of the bile in the liver.
Consultant	That's right. The bilirubin released from the red cells in haemolytic jaundice has not been conjugated in the liver and so it is not water-soluble and can't therefore be dissolved and excreted in the urine. You do, however, get an excess of urobilinogen in the urine. What about hepatocellular jaundice, or as it is called nowadays, cholestatic jaundice — what are the urinary findings in this condition?
Student	The bilirubin has been through the liver and been conjugated, so it can appear in the urine and make it dark.
Consultant	What about the stools in cholestatic jaundice?
Student	They could be paler than normal.
Consultant	They are usually pale in this type of jaundice but the degree of pallor will obviously depend on the severity of obstruction of the bile canaliculi inside the liver. Let us return now to clinical matters. Can you think of any other conditions that can cause pale stools?
Student	The stools tend to be pale in any case of severe diarrhoea.
Consultant	There is one particular type of diarrhoea I have in mind.
Student	Do you mean malabsorption?
Consultant	I do indeed. Does she have malabsorption?
Student	She could do. Don't you get malabsorption as a result of obstructive jaundice?
Consultant	That is physiologically true but malabsorption is not usually a significant clinical complication of obstructive jaundice. Let me ask you again whether Mrs S. has malabsorption?
Student	She will need specific investigations to find out.
Consultant	Can't you find out by asking her some simple questions?
Student	I forgot to ask her about the nature of her stools, and in particular, whether they are bulky, offensive and difficult to flush away.
Consultant	Would you like to ask her now?
Student	Mrs S., do you have any difficulty in flushing away your motions in the toilet — do they cling to the toilet bowl?
Patient	I can't say that I've ever noticed any difficulty. The motions seem to flush away quite easily.
Consultant	That tells us she is very unlikely to have malabsorption. I think that we have established that Mrs S. has obstructive jaundice and I'd like you to tell me what you think are the possible causes. Now, before you start, I don't want you to reel off the usual list of causes of obstructive jaundice that you find in the textbooks — I want you to relate the possible causes directly to Mrs S.'s history.

Student	I think that the first diagnosis to consider is gallbladder disease, because she gives a long history of flatulent dyspepsia and she has been jaundiced before.
Consultant	Contrary to widespread, and misplaced, belief flatulent dyspepsia is not indicative of chronic gallbladder disease. It occurs as frequently in patients without gallbladder trouble as with chronic gallbladder disease; furthermore, if a patient with proven gallbladder disease and flatulent dyspepsia has a cholecystectomy the dyspepsia almost always persists.
	The most likely cause of so-called flatulent dyspepsia is irritable bowel syndrome, but I don't want to be diverted onto that subject at the moment.
	If Mrs S.'s first attack of jaundice had been due to gallbladder disease, she would most likely have had severe pain either from acute cholecystitis or from an impacted gallstone or both.
	Did she have severe pain with the first attack of jaundice?
Student	I'm sorry I didn't ask, but I'll ask her now.
Patient	No, I can't remember any really severe pain in my stomach when I was jaundiced, but it was uncomfortable in the upper part and my GP said it was over my liver.
Consultant	What does that suggest to you?
Student	It sounds as if she may have had hepatitis.
Consultant	I would agree with you — we'll come back to that later.
	Can you think of any other possible causes of her present jaundice?
Student	You must always consider a neoplasm.
Consultant	A good suggestion! We must certainly consider this possibility when jaundice occurs in middle age. Where would you think would be the likely site?
Student	It could be in the pancreas.
Consultant	Yes, that is one of the commonest sites in obstructive jaundice. Anywhere else?
Student	The jaundice may be the result of direct involvement of the liver itself by neoplasm.
Consultant	Metastatic deposits in the liver are a possible cause, as well as involvement of the glands in the porta hepatis with compression of the common bile duct leading to obstructive jaundice.
	Is there any support in the history for the diagnosis of neoplasm?
Student	There are two relevant symptoms — she has lost her appetite and she is also losing weight.
Consultant	These may well be relevant symptoms in this particular diagnosis and we will have to keep it in mind. Can you think of any other possible causes for the jaundice?
Student	The other diagnosis which occurs to me is cirrhosis of the liver.

Consultant	What type of cirrhosis?
Student	The commonest type is alcoholic cirrhosis.
Consultant	I don't dispute that, but it's not very likely in Mrs S. is it since she doesn't drink, or at least drinks very little, so what other type of cirrhosis would you suggest?
Student	The other possibility is biliary cirrhosis.
Consultant	That's more like it. Biliary cirrhosis, as you will no doubt remember, can be either secondary to gallbladder disease or primary which is probably an auto-immune disease. This diagnosis also remains a possibility. Any other causes of cirrhosis?
Student	Wilson's* disease.
Consultant	That's a very rare condition. Do you know the cause?
Student	I think it's something to do with copper.
Consultant	Wilson's disease, or hepato-lenticular degeneration, is due to an abnormality of copper metabolism which results in the deposition of copper in various organs including the liver and basal ganglia. It is a congenital condition and I think highly unlikely in Mrs S.
	Can you think of any other causes of cirrhosis?
Student	Apart from idiopathic cirrhosis, I can't think of any more.
Consultant	'Idiopathic' means we don't know the cause so it's not really a very helpful diagnosis, is it?
	Is diabetes associated with cirrhosis?
Student	Not that I know of.
Consultant	Have you ever heard of 'bronze' diabetes?
Student	You mean haemochromatosis.
Consultant	Good. What are the features of this condition?
Student	You get a combination of cirrhosis and diabetes. I think it's due to excessive deposition of iron in the tissues.
Consultant	That's quite right. It is due to an abnormality of iron metabolism with excessive absorption of iron into the circulation. Apart from cirrhosis and diabetes, the other clinical features are a slaty-grey pigmentation, testicular atrophy with loss of axillary hair, polyarthropathy and heart failure. I think we will both agree that Mrs S. is not a man, and since this disorder occurs almost exclusively in men, it is very unlikely that Mrs S. has haemochromatosis.
	The final cause we ought to consider is chronic hepatitis. Do you know anything about this?

* S.A.K. Wilson (1877–1937) was an American who qualified in Edinburgh and became a neurologist at the National Hospital for Nervous Diseases in Queen's Square. He published his MD thesis on 'Progressive lenticular degeneration: a familial nervous disease associated with cirrhosis of the liver'.

Student	I know that chronic hepatitis can be either active or passive, and it can sometimes follow acute hepatitis.
Consultant	As you say, chronic hepatitis can be either passive, or to be more accurate, persistent which may show very little in the way of symptoms, or it can be chronic active or aggressive hepatitis which carries a much worse prognosis.
	Both the persistent and active type can follow acute hepatitis type B, or possibly non A-non B hepatitis, but is extremely rare after type A hepatitis. Chronic active hepatitis probably occurs in 5–10% of patients after hepatitis type B. Do you think this is relevant in Mrs S.?
Student	Yes, it could well be. Mrs S. did have an attack of jaundice 5 years ago which was associated with pain over the liver which could well have been acute hepatitis type B.
Consultant	That is certainly a possibility, but we would need some more information before deciding that Mrs S. had hepatitis B, such as whether she had any injections or blood transfusions, or had she taken 'main-line' drugs.
Student	I'm sorry, I haven't asked her any of those questions.
Patient	(Indignantly) I've never been a drug addict!
Consultant	Please forgive me, Mrs S., for mentioning the drugs and I certainly know that it doesn't apply to you. I'm only trying to help our young friend here to learn. (To student) Are there any other possible causes of chronic active hepatitis which might be applicable to Mrs S.?
Student	Not that I can think of.
Consultant	Chronic active hepatitis can occur with some hepatotoxic drugs of which one is methyldopa (Aldomet). Mrs S. is being treated for hypertension — is she taking methyldopa?
Student	She can't remember the name of the tablets she is taking for her blood pressure.
Consultant	Mrs S., are the tablets yellow and fairly large?
Patient	Yes, they are.
Consultant	Then it is possible that she is taking methyldopa and we must keep this in mind as a possible relevant factor in causing the jaundice. Are there any other drugs she is taking which might be hepatotoxic?
Student	I think that diazepam can sometimes damage the liver.
Consultant	Yes, it can, though in my experience it is rare. The type of liver damage with diazepam leads to cholestatic jaundice, unlike methyldopa where the damage affects the liver cells directly and can sometimes end with chronic active hepatitis. Is there anything else in Mrs S.'s history which might support the diagnosis of chronic active hepatitis?
Student	I don't think so.

Consultant	What about the pain in her joints?
Student	I didn't know that joint pain was a symptom of the condition.
Consultant	Polyarthritis is an extra-hepatic complication of chronic active hepatitis. Do you know of any other conditions which may occur with chronic active hepatitis?
Student	I can't think of anything else.
Consultant	Chronic active hepatitis is an auto-immune disease and may therefore be associated with other auto-immune diseases such as rheumatoid arthritis, glomerulonephritis, ulcerative colitis or Crohn's* disease, and Hashimoto's[†] thyroiditis.
	What about the family history — do you think this might have a bearing on Mrs S.'s problems?
Student	Her sister has rheumatoid arthritis and in the light of what we have just been saying, this could well be relevant.
Consultant	We seem to be building up quite a case in favour of chronic active hepatitis.
	I think that we have probably got most of the important diagnostic clues from the history, so perhaps we can now summarize our conclusions:

HISTORY

- we consider that Mrs S. has obstructive jaundice
- she may have had an attack of acute hepatitis previously which could have gone on to chronic active hepatitis
- she is probably taking two possibly hepatotoxic drugs — diazepam and methyldopa — which may also be relevant in causing her jaundice
- the anorexia and the loss of weight raises the possibility of neoplastic disease, and the two likely organs involved are the pancreas and the liver
- Mrs S.'s polyarthritis and the family history of rheumatoid arthritis supports the diagnosis of chronic active hepatitis

---

Consultant	And now I'd like you to tell us your examination findings. Remember the problem we're dealing with is jaundice and we have discussed the likely causes so I want you to present your findings with these possible diagnoses in mind (Figure 7.1).

* B.B. Crohn (1884–1983) was an American gastroenterologist who worked at the Mount Sinai Hospital in New York.
[†] H. Hashimoto (1881–1934) was a Japanese surgeon who wrote his MD thesis on 'Struma lymphomatosa' while working in the surgical department of Kyushu University.

Student	The first thing to note is that she is jaundiced and she has some scratch marks on her skin which confirms our view that the jaundice is obstructive. I've also noticed that she has bruises on her legs and she told me that as far as she can remember she didn't injure her legs to cause the bruises.
Consultant	What do you deduce from this point?
Student	That she has spontaneous bruising which is probably due to the lack of absorption of vitamin K as a result of the obstructive jaundice — this will lower the prothrombin concentration in the blood and as a result spontaneous bleeding can occur.
Consultant	You have explained that very well. There is of course another possible factor to account for the tendency to bleed, isn't there?
Student	I don't know.
Consultant	Liver damage itself can lead to defective synthesis of prothrombin, and in very severe cases, fibrinogen as well. How would we decide whether the problem is failure of absorption of vitamin K or defective hepatic synthesis?
Student	By giving her an injection of vitamin K and seeing whether it increases the prothrombin concentration in the blood.
Consultant	That's right — it is a very useful test. Please go on with your examination.
Student	She doesn't have any enlarged neck glands.
Consultant	Why do you mention that?
Student	To exclude a neoplasm in the abdomen as we considered earlier in the differential diagnosis of the jaundice.
Consultant	Don't forget reticulosis as another possible cause of lymphadenopathy. Go on.
Student	The pulse was 68/minute and regular, the blood pressure was 180/110, the apex beat was normal and I thought the heart was normal with no murmurs.
Consultant	All valid observations I have no doubt, but I would have preferred you to follow up your original observations about the jaundice and the glands by commenting on findings relevant to the main problem which relates primarily to liver disease.
Student	She does have an enlarged liver.
Consultant	Could you give us a little more detail about the liver?
Student	It was about 3 cm below the costal margin with a firm, smooth surface and no nodules or irregularity. It was slightly tender.
Consultant	Were there any other relevant abdominal findings?
Student	I couldn't feel the spleen and there were no other abdominal masses palpable.

Consultant	Any ascites?
Student	No, and I did check.
Consultant	Good, anything else interesting to show us?
Student	No, I don't think so.
Consultant	What about signs of cirrhosis? Have you any comments about her finger nails, palms and superficial abdominal veins; also does she have any spider naevi?
Student	I did look at her nails and wondered whether they could be clubbed. I didn't notice any spider naevi. She doesn't have a caput medusae.
Consultant	Every student mentions the caput medusae.* I've never seen one in cirrhosis. You are much more likely to get distended superficial abdominal veins running vertically from the groin up to the umbilicus. What does it signify?
Student	It would show that there is a blockage in the portal circulation so that the splanchnic blood flow is diverted to the systemic venous circulation and therefore bypasses the liver.
Consultant	Do you think that bypassing the liver carries any particular hazards?
Student	Yes, it means that there would be toxic substances passing into the systemic circulation which would normally be detoxicated in the liver.
Consultant	Do you know what clinical effects these toxic agents might have on the patient?
Student	They could cause hepatic encephalopathy.
Consultant	Good. Does Mrs S. show any evidence of this?
Student	I'm sorry I didn't test for this as I didn't think of this complication.
Consultant	I think it is always wise to keep this in mind in any jaundiced patient — I find it is often forgotten! Would you like to test for it now — that is if you know how?

The student asks the patient to stretch out her hands in front of her and reports that there is no 'flap'.

Consultant	Holding out the arms is a good screening test for hepatic failure. Other parts of the nervous system can also be involved, especially the pyramidal tracts, so don't forget to carry out a more detailed neurological examination if a hepatic flap is present. A patient's hands can tell you a lot about the liver. I agree that she has finger clubbing which is a sign of cirrhosis. Do you know any other sign in the finger nails?

* Medusa in classical mythology was the chief of the Gorgons whose hair was transformed into a mass of writhing serpents and whose face was so terrible to behold that all who looked on it were transformed into stone.

Student	No, I can't think of any.
Consultant	You may get white bands across the nail in cirrhosis which is thought to be caused by periods of reduced protein synthesis. What about her palms?
Student	They look normal to me.
Consultant	I don't agree. Don't you think that there is a distinct pinker area on the medial side of both palms?
Student	Now you have pointed it out to me I would agree.
Consultant	What is its significance?
Student	I think it's because of high levels of circulating oestrogen.
Consultant	That is the generally accepted view though it is open to some doubt when you try to prove it by measurement. It is said to be due to lack of breakdown of the oestrogens by the diseased liver producing excessive dilatation of capillaries. Spider naevi are thought to have the same origin. There is one other manifestation of liver disease in the hands — do you know what it is?
Student	Is it Dupuytren's contracture?*
Consultant	That's right. It is found particularly in alcoholic liver disease. Now, I should like to turn to the possible causes of the liver enlargement. Do you have any ideas about this?
Student	I don't think it is neoplastic.
Consultant	Why not?
Student	Because the liver is too smooth — there are no irregular areas which might indicate metastases.
Consultant	What are the other possibilities then?
Student	It could be cirrhosis.
Consultant	What kind of cirrhosis do you have in mind?
Student	It could be due to alcohol or it may be chronic active hepatitis as we mentioned in the history.
Consultant	You have already pointed out that Mrs S. drinks very little alcohol so this diagnosis is excluded, but I would agree that chronic active hepatitis remains a likely possibility. Any other causes of cirrhosis worth mentioning?
Student	Biliary cirrhosis is another possible diagnosis.
Consultant	Yes, we were discussing this when we talked about the history. You will remember that biliary cirrhosis can be caused either by gallbladder

---

* Baron G. Dupuytren (1777–1835) was Professor of Operative Surgery in the famous French Hospital, the Hôtel-Dieu, in Paris and was chief surgeon to the French King, Charles X.

disease or it can be primary. Do you know any other name for primary biliary cirrhosis?

Student No, I'm sorry I don't, but I would guess that you are going to come up with another eponymous name.

Consultant Good for you! I'm glad that you are beginning to anticipate my methods — it might stand you in good stead if you are able to do the same with your examiners! Primary biliary cirrhosis is also called Hanot's* cirrhosis. Do you know any signs on examination which might help you in making this diagnosis?

Student I think that the patient may have a high cholesterol in this condition.

Consultant That's right, and what do you think this might lead to in the way of signs?

Student She might develop xanthomata.

Consultant She could indeed develop cholesterol deposits in the skin and tendons, and also around the eyes which we call . . . ?

Student Xanthelasma.

Consultant I think we should now consider the rest of your examination findings. Did you find anything else of interest?

Student I've already given you the findings in the cardiovascular system and the only abnormality was the hypertension. The lungs were clear.

I realize now that I haven't examined the nervous system in as much detail as I should have done — all I checked were the pupils and the reflexes and these appeared to be normal.

Consultant I'm afraid that there is an unfortunate tendency to do only a cursory examination of the nervous sytem during a routine clinical examination, and I'm often pained to hear phrases like 'The nervous sytem was grossly normal' — translated, this usually means 'I only carried out a token check of the pupils and knee jerks' — findings which are really of negligible value on their own. And when students write down phrases like CNS — n.a.d, I sometimes wonder whether what is really meant is 'not actually done'.

Anything else on examination?

Student I think we have covered everything.

Consultant There is one other thing that you have missed out — whether Mrs S. has any of the other auto-immune conditions which may be associated with chronic active hepatitis; you remember we mentioned them earlier. Would you like to remind us what they were?

Student Arthritis and ulcerative colitis or Crohn's disease.

* V.C. Hanot (1844–1896) was a French physician who described biliary cirrhosis in 1875. He was a colleague of the great French neurologist, Jean Charcot.

Consultant	Also glomerulonephritis and Hashimoto's thyroiditis.
Student	I don't think that there was evidence of any of these conditions on examination.
Consultant	No, I agree that Mrs S. does not have any of these disorders — the important thing is to think of them all in any patient with an auto-immune disease and to make sure you look for them. Now, I think we have exhausted the clinical findings, so let's summarize our conclusions as we should always do at the end of the examination:

> EXAMINATION
>
> - we have confirmed the obstructive jaundice by the scratch marks
> - she has smooth hepatic enlargement which we don't think is likely to be neoplastic
> - there is impairment of hepatic function as indicated by the pink palms and the spontaneous bruising
> - there is no evidence of hepatic encephalopathy
> - we consider that chronic active hepatitis remains a likely diagnosis, and there is no clinical evidence of any other associated auto-immune disorder

Consultant	Let us now discuss the investigations which will help us to diagnose Mrs S.'s jaundice. How are you going to approach this?
Student	I think we should first try to confirm the type of jaundice by examining her urine.
Consultant	I'm glad you have started with this simple and very helpful test in a case of jaundice. What would you look for in the urine?
Student	For bile pigments.
Consultant	Which ones are you interested in?
Student	Bilirubin and urobilinogen.
Consultant	How would these help you?
Student	In obstructive jaundice you would get an excess of both bilirubin and urobilinogen in the urine.
Consultant	That's right but remember the urobilinogen would only be present if the obstruction wasn't complete, otherwise the urobilinogen would be absent altogether from the urine. What would you think of if you had a jaundiced patient with no bilirubin in the urine?
Student	It would suggest haemolytic jaundice.
Consultant	In this case the excess of bilirubin in the circulation causing the jaundice is of the pre-hepatic or unconjugated type where the molecules are insoluble in water and as a result are unable to be excreted in the urine.

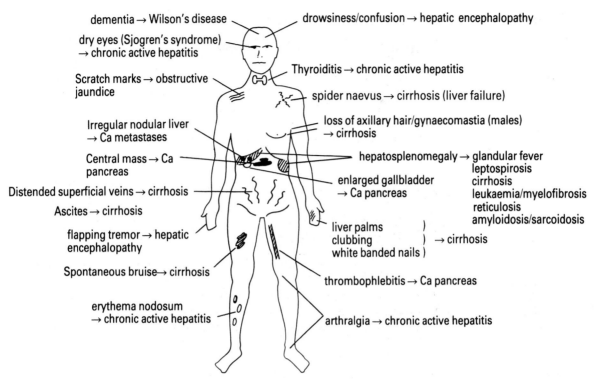

Figure 7.1 Possible helpful diagnostic signs in a patient with jaundice.

Here is Mrs S.'s urine result. There is an excess of both bilirubin and urobilinogen — what are your comments?

Student   She has obstructive jaundice and the obstruction is not complete.

Consultant   What test would you like to do next?

Student   I think the next investigation should be liver function tests.

Consultant   Yes, this is also a necessary test in a jaundiced patient. Let me show you Mrs S.'s results.

		Normal range
Bilirubin	57 mmol/L	5–17
Alk. phosphatase	520 units/L	102–289
Gamma-GT	187 units/L	6–42
Albumin	31.5 g/L	35–50
AST	87 units/L	5–35
ALT	59 units/L	5–35

What do you think these results indicate?

Student	They confirm the jaundice and they also indicate liver cell damage.
Consultant	More specifically, the increased bilirubin confirms the jaundice, the raised alkaline phosphatase shows cholestasis (stasis of bile), the increased gamma-GT and raised transaminases indicate liver cell damage and the low albumin shows impaired protein synthesis. What's the next test?
Student	We could investigate the possibility of hepatitis.
Consultant	The tests you mean are serum tests for infection with hepatitis A, B and non A-non B. Do you think these tests would be very relevant to Mrs S.'s problems?
Student	I don't think that Mrs S. has infective hepatitis at the moment, but if the test was positive for hepatitis it might support the possibility of chronic active hepatitis, since you pointed out earlier that chronic hepatitis may sometimes follow hepatitis B.
Consultant	That's good reasoning. We are currently awaiting the results of Mrs S.'s serum tests for hepatitis so we can't tell you the result yet. What other tests do we need to do?
Student	How about radiology?
Consultant	What do you want to X-ray?
Student	We could do a cholecystogram.
Consultant	And what would we be looking for in the cholecystogram?
Student	It might show gallstones or a non-functioning gallbladder which could have led to biliary cirrhosis.
Consultant	OK I'll accept that answer though I could perhaps remind you that there was nothing in the history to suggest previous gallbladder disease. Additionally, the gallbladder is unlikely to show well or even at all in a cholecystogram in a jaundiced patient since the dye will not be excreted adequately. If you are looking for gallstones in a jaundiced patient it is always worth thinking of a simple straight X-ray of the abdomen, since about 30% of gallstones are radio-opaque — here is an example of a cholecystogram in another patient that I had (Figure 7.2). Apart from this simple X-ray of the abdomen, there is another radiological test which can be used; it is also of value if the gallbladder is not functioning or has been removed — do you know what it is?
Student	The only other X-ray I can think of is intravenous cholangiography.
Consultant	That is the test I had in mind. It is useful also if you suspect a stone in the common bile duct. I don't think it would be of much help in Mrs S. Can you think of any other tests?
Student	What about abdominal ultrasound?
Consultant	Abdominal ultrasound is perhaps the most useful test of all in a patient with obstructive jaundice. Do you know why I say that?

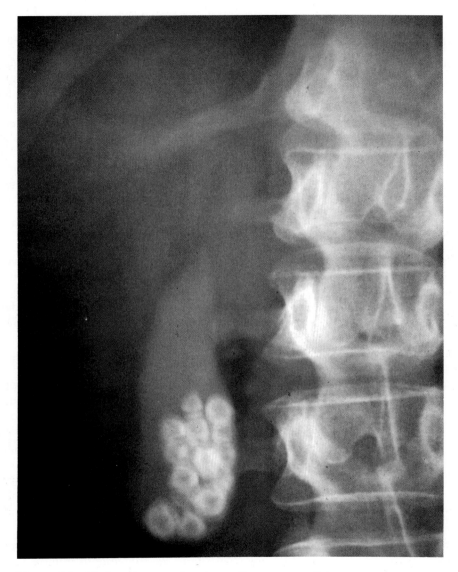

Figure 7.2 Cholecystogram showing radio-opaque gallstones.

Student	It could show an irregular liver due to cirrhosis or it may show neoplastic deposits.
Consultant	That is quite true, but the reason I stressed the value of this test in obstructive jaundice is that it helps to decide whether the jaundice has a medical origin or a surgical cause. Do you know how?
Student	I think that it depends on the dilatation of the intra-hepatic ducts.
Consultant	That is quite right. If the intra-hepatic ducts are widely dilated then it is likely to be a surgical problem: the sizes usually given are >4 mm in diameter for the common hepatic duct and >7 mm for the common bile duct. If this degree of dilatation is present then it is likely that the patient has extra-hepatic obstruction, the most frequent causes of which are gallstones, carcinoma of the pancreas or enlarged glands in the porta hepatis. Mrs S. showed mild enlargement of the liver and no dilatation of the bile ducts so she is unlikely to have mechanical obstruction of the bile ducts. What test should we do next?
Student	I think that the quickest way of getting an answer in Mrs S. is going to be a liver biopsy.
Consultant	And I would agree with you. Before you do the liver biopsy, however, you must always check first that there is no bleeding tendency due to prothrombin deficiency resulting from the liver disease — if there is, you must correct it with vitamin K injections before undertaking the biopsy. What might you find in Mrs S.'s liver biopsy if she had chronic active hepatitis?
Student	All I remember is that you can get areas of necrosis.
Consultant	The type of necrosis that you find is called 'piecemeal necrosis' which means areas of hepatocyte destruction distributed randomly through the hepatic lobule. Other distinctive histological features include 'rosettes' of regenerating liver cells, fibrous bridges and infiltration with plasma cells and lymphocytes (Figure 7.3). Mrs S.'s liver biopsy showed the typical features of chronic active hepatitis. Are there any other tests which might help to diagnose this condition?
Student	I think that you can get anti-bodies in the blood but I can't remember the details of which ones.
Consultant	The test we do for anti-bodies is the collagen screen. The anti-bodies we look for particularly are the smooth muscle and anti-mitochondrial anti-bodies. In chronic active hepatitis smooth muscle anti-bodies are present in 40–80% while anti-mitochondrial anti-bodies are infrequent, perhaps only 10–20%: this contrasts with primary biliary cirrhosis where anti-mitochondrial anti-bodies are found in 90% and smooth muscle anti-bodies are much less frequent; another anti-body which is present in 25–50% of patients with chronic active hepatitis is anti-nuclear factor.

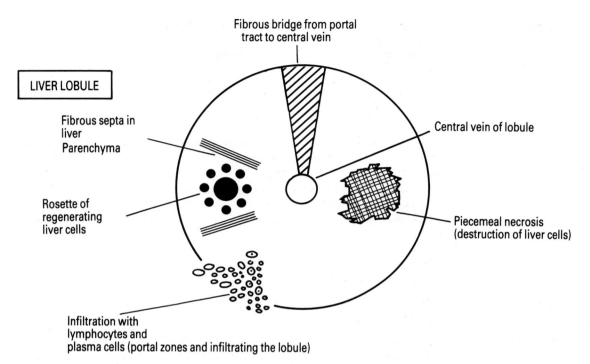

Fibrous bridge from portal
tract to central vein

LIVER LOBULE

Fibrous septa in
liver
Parenchyma

Central vein of lobule

Rosette of
regenerating
liver cells

Piecemeal necrosis
(destruction of liver cells)

Infiltration with
lymphocytes and
plasma cells (portal zones and infiltrating the lobule)

Figure 7.3 Diagram of histological changes in liver biopsy of chronic active hepatitis.

Here is the result of Mrs S.'s anti-body screen:

Smooth muscle anti-body	40
Mitochondrial	nil
Anti-nuclear	100

The first thing to say is that the absence of anti-mitochondrial anti-bodies excludes primary biliary cirrhosis in Mrs S., which you might well have thought of in the light of her age and sex, itching, obstructive jaundice and high alkaline phosphatase.

These findings are strongly suggestive of chronic active hepatitis.

The other important test in chronic active hepatitis is an increase in IgG level — Mrs S. showed 19 g/L compared with a normal level of 6 – 16 g/L.

We have now confirmed the diagnosis of chronic active hepatitis in Mrs S. Perhaps we can now briefly consider treatment. What are your views on this?

Student   I think that we ought to consider a course of steroids, because chronic active hepatitis may be an auto-immune disease and therefore should respond to steroids.

Consultant	I would agree with you. Chronic active hepatitis may indeed be of auto-immune origin but don't forget it can also be drug-induced or follow hepatitis B. Can you tell clinically whether the condition is of the auto-immune type?
Student	I don't think so — you need the results of the tests.
Consultant	You can get some help from the clinical history as well. Mrs S. does have a family history of probable auto-immune disease — her sister has rheumatoid arthritis — and Mrs S. herself has polyarthralgia which could well be an auto-immune extra-hepatic manifestation of chronic active hepatitis.

If you really want to be scientific, however, one of the most useful indications of potential responsiveness is the liver biopsy — if bridging necrosis is present there is a strong chance of progression to cirrhosis, and in these circumstances, prednisolone is indicated to prevent this progression.

If there is no bridging necrosis then the prognosis is likely to be good and steroids are not necessary.

Since Mrs S. does show bridging necrosis in her liver biopsy we will treat her with prednisolone, starting with 60 mg daily, then tapering to a maintenance dose of 20 mg daily within a few weeks. We shall assess her progress clinically and repeat the liver biopsy in about six months to get a more accurate idea of her response.

OUTCOME

Mrs S. responded satisfactorily to treatment with the prednisolone. Her jaundice steadily improved, her appetite returned to normal and her weight loss stopped over a period of several weeks. A repeat liver biopsy 6 months later showed histological improvement with less bridging necrosis and an increase in the extent of the regenerating 'rosettes'. She was able to reduce the maintenance dose of prednisolone to 7.5 mg daily and on this dose was entirely free of side-effects over the period of follow-up which to date amounted to 4 years.

NB The auto-immune type of chronic active hepatitis carries a less favourable prognosis than that following hepatitis B, with a 50–75% mortality within the first few years.

This type of chronic active hepatitis usually affects young women, whereas the cases following hepatitis B usually occur in older men and are diagnosed by finding the blood is HB_sAg-positive.

LEARNING POINTS

Urinary bile pigments in differentiating jaundice

	Haemolytic	*Hepato-cellular*	*Obstructive*
Bilirubin	—	++	++
Urobilinogen	++	++	—

Significance of liver function tests

- bilirubin → degree of jaundice
- alkaline phosphatase → intrahepatic cholestasis
- transaminases → liver cell damage
- albumin → synthesis of protein

Causes of hepato-splenomegaly

- infection
    glandular fever
    leptospirosis
- cirrhosis
- reticulosis
- amyloidosis
- sarcoidosis
- chronic leukaemia
- myelofibrosis

Hepato-toxic drugs

- psychotropic
    monoamine-oxidase inhibitors
    tricyclic antidepressives
    phenothiazines
    benzodiazepines
- non-steroidal anti-inflammatory drugs
- gold and penicillamine
- anti-hypertensives
    methyldopa
    hydralazine
- anti-diabetic
    chlorpropamide
    tolbutamide
- anti-convulsants
    phenytoin
- anti-biotics
    sulphonamides
    nitrofurantoin
    isoniazid

Drugs causing cholestatic jaundice

- tricyclic anti-depressives
- phenothiazines
- benzodiazepines
- gold
- chlorpropamide, tolbutamide
- oral contraceptives

Drugs causing chronic active hepatitis

- isoniazid
- nitrofurantoin
- dantrolene
- methyldopa

Causes of obstructive (cholestatic) jaundice

large ducts
- gallstones
- carcinoma of pancreas
- carcinoma of Ampulla of Vater*
- glands in the porta hepatis

small ducts
- cirrhosis
- drugs — tricyclic anti-depressives
         phenothiazines
         benzodiazepines
         chlorpropamide
         tolbutamide
         oral contraceptives
         gold
- reticulosis
- liver metastases

Causes of cirrhosis

- alcohol
- biliary
    primary
    secondary to gallbladder disease
- chronic hepatitis
    persistent
    active (aggressive)
- haemachromatosis

* A. Vater (1684–1751) was a German anatomist who became Professor of Medicine at Wittenberg.

- Wilson's disease (hepato-lenticular degeneration)
- idiopathic — cause unknown

Differentiation between primary biliary cirrhosis and chronic active hepatitis

	Primary biliary cirrhosis	*Chronic active hepatitis*
Pruritus	frequent	variable
Xanthelasma	+	±
Serum cholesterol	raised	normal
Alkaline phosphatase	raised ++	normal or +
Serum anti-bodies	anti-mitochondrial	anti-smooth muscle

Signs of hepatic encephalopathy

- foetor hepaticus
- flapping tremor
- drowsiness/confusion
- slurred speech
- pyramidal signs
- (raised blood ammonia level)

Factors influencing decision on steroid treatment in chronic active hepatitis

- presence of symptoms
- age and sex (young females especially)
- auto-immune features evident
- HB$_s$Ag status (negative)
- bridging necrosis in liver biopsy

8

Headache

Student

Mrs N.D. is a 55-year-old teacher who was well until about 3 months ago when she started to get increasing trouble with her migraine. She has suffered with attacks of migraine since she was 15 years old and the attacks continued to give her problems until her late twenties and then appeared to subside. She has had an occasional attack since, usually when she has been under stress. She has had a lot of stress over the past few months because she is going through a divorce and she thinks that is the reason why the migraine has returned. She has been getting headaches almost every day and they often make her feel sick — in fact she has vomited when the headache has been bad as she used to do in her teens. The other symptom she has noticed is her vision 'goes a bit funny' when she has the headache, and this always used to happen with her migraine attacks in the past when she used to go partially blind with the headaches.

On systematic enquiry, she has not had any fits and has not noticed any weakness of her limbs though she did mention some tingling in her left leg occasionally but she thinks that she has probably had this for years as she has suffered with a slipped disc in the past causing sciatica in the left leg. She admitted to a smoker's cough which she has had for years — she smokes 15 cigarettes a day usually though she said she has been smoking more recently because of her divorce. There was nothing else relevant in the other systems on direct enquiry.

In the past history, apart from the migraine and the sciatica which I've already mentioned, she is also being treated for high blood pressure which she has had since her daughter was born 22 years ago — she had toxaemia of pregnancy — and she is currently on atenolol 100 mg daily.

There is a family history of hypertension; her father had high blood pressure and died of a stroke at the age of 67, and she has a brother who is also being treated for high blood pressure. There is no history of migraine in the family.

Mrs D. drinks very little alcohol — she has always avoided drinking because it makes her migraine worse.

Consultant

Would you like to try to analyse the history for us at this stage and point us towards some possible diagnoses?

Student	Mrs D.'s main symptom is the headache and the most likely diagnosis I think is a severe recurrence of the migraine which she thinks herself is probably brought on by all the recent emotional trauma of her divorce.
Consultant	Yes, obviously this is a possibility, though — with every respect for Mrs D.'s opinion — it is wise not to be unduly influenced by the patient's views on the diagnosis. I hasten to add that you should always pay attention to what the patient thinks as I have come across occasions when the patient has been right and the doctor — including myself — has been wrong. I remember a young and very anxious man with persistent headache which had all the classical features of a tension headache — I hope we shall be going over these features shortly — but neither he nor his family would accept this diagnosis. They were sure that he had something seriously wrong with him. Unusually for tension headache, the symptoms remained unchanged in spite of adequate reassurance and eventually a CT scan was arranged — this showed a very rare type of space-occupying lesion of the corpus callosum. This helped to teach me to be very wary of dismissing patients' views. What causes other than migraine might you consider to account for Mrs D.'s headaches?
Student	She could have tension headache in view of all the emotional trauma that she has been going through.
Consultant	OK, this certainly should be included in the differential diagnosis.
Student	We should also consider the possibility of a space-occupying lesion in the brain, especially in the light of your recent comments.
Consultant	Yes, this diagnosis should always be thought of in any late-onset headache. Any other possible causes?
Student	The other possibility that occurs to me is that the headache might be related to her high blood pressure.
Consultant	You're doing very well. You have mentioned most of the relevant diagnoses. Perhaps we might consider each diagnosis in a little more detail now. It's very important to remember that the diagnosis in most cases of headache is made primarily on the history and the nature of the headache, including the site, timing, character, aggravating and relieving factors and associated symptoms. What can you tell us now about Mrs D.'s headache in relation to the features we've just mentioned and does it help us in deciding the cause?
Student	The site of Mrs D.'s headache is sometimes in the front over her eyes and sometimes at the back of her head. She also said that it was usually a thumping headache.
Consultant	What is your interpretation of these factors?
Student	A thumping headache is very suggestive of migraine.
Consultant	I agree. What about the varying site?

Student	I think that you can get migrainous headache in various parts of the head.
Consultant	In 'classic' migraine the headache can vary in site but is almost always unilateral, so this is not like 'classic' migraine. You can get a generalized throbbing headache in so-called 'common migraine', which often occurs at weekends and in women in the premenstrual period. Basilar migraine, which is rare, can cause occipital headache. So far, then, Mrs D. might have common or basilar migraine. Can you tell us anything about the timing of the headache?
Student	I'm sorry I forgot to ask, but I'll ask her now. Mrs D., does the headache occur at any particular time of the day?
Patient	I haven't noticed any special time of the day when I get the headache, it can occur any time and can sometimes go on all day.
Consultant	Have you got all the information you want on the timing now?
Student	I think so. It doesn't seem to have any particular pattern during the day.
Consultant	Don't you think it would be important to know whether Mrs D. gets the headache during the night as well as the day?
Student	Yes, of course, I should have asked her this. Mrs D. do you ever get the headache at night in bed?
Patient	Yes, I have been waking in the night with quite severe headache and have sometimes been sick with it.
Consultant	Mrs D., have you ever awakened in the morning with the headache?
Patient	Yes, I have. This is worrying me because it seems to be getting more frequent now.
Consultant	What do you make of this?
Student	Headache in the night and also on waking in the morning occurs with space-occupying lesions of the brain.
Consultant	Right, but hypertensive headache can also be similar, so let's keep both these possibilities in mind. Are there any aggravating or relieving factors?
Student	Mrs D. says that stress brings on her headaches.
Consultant	That occurs particularly in migraine. Any other aggravating factors?
Student	I should have asked her about the effect of straining.
Consultant	Why?
Student	Because this can make headache worse if raised intracranial pressure is present.
Consultant	That's right. Would you like to ask her about this?
Student	Mrs D., do you find that straining makes your headache worse.
Consultant	If I may interject before Mrs D. answers you. That type of leading question would never be allowed in a court of law, so I don't think we should

	allow it here. You should ask her whether straining affects her headache in any way, either to make it better or worse.
Student	Mrs D., have you noticed whether straining has any effect on your headache, either to make it better or worse?
Consultant	That's much better. Would you answer the student's question please, Mrs D.?
Patient	What do you mean by straining, doctor?
Consultant	By straining, we mean making a severe physical effort, for example if you are constipated and you are straining hard to pass your motion.
Patient	I'm not sure about the effect of straining but what I have noticed is that bending down or coughing always seems to give me more headache.
Consultant	Thank you Mrs D., that's an important observation. (Addressing the student) That brings us back to the likelihood of raised intracranial pressure. You said she vomited with the headache; what is the relevance of this?
Student	Vomiting can occur both in migraine and with raised intracranial pressure so it doesn't really help to distinguish between the two.
Consultant	It would help if you could tell us whether the vomiting brings the headache to an end, as in migraine, or has no effect on the headache.
Student	I'm sorry I didn't ask her about that. Mrs D., is the headache relieved when you vomit, or perhaps I'd better ask you whether vomiting has any effect on the headache, then it won't be a leading question.
Patient	When I used to get migraine I found that the attack would always end when I vomited. The recent headaches seem different, and now the vomiting doesn't relieve it, in fact it makes it worse.
Consultant	I think we can gather from what Mrs D. has so clearly said, that the headache and vomiting that she gets now is unlikely to be due to migraine. What about hypertensive headache?
Student	No, it can't be this because I found her blood pressure was normal when I checked it.
Consultant	That may be so, but it's no answer to the question. You will remember that we are analysing the history, so we must base our judgement on the symptoms and not on any signs that you may have found on your examination. What I'm really getting at are the features of hypertensive headache.
Student	It's a severe headache which affects the frontal area and, as you mentioned earlier, it can occur at night as well as on waking in the morning.
Consultant	That's right, apart from the site — it is usually occipital and not frontal. What about the character?
Student	It's a throbbing headache.

Consultant	Yes, a throbbing headache always suggests a vascular origin, apart, perhaps, from a special condition in which the blood vessels are affected and the headache tends to be a constant burning or boring pain — do you know what I have in mind?
Student	No, I'm sorry.
Consultant	I'm thinking of temporal arteritis, though the same features would occur with arteritis elsewhere; also in migrainous neuralgia, otherwise called cluster headache, the pain is not throbbing but burning or piercing.

On the basis of the headache alone, we would not therefore be able to exclude hypertensive headache in Mrs D.

Now before we leave the question of the differential diagnosis of headache, I think we should just mention the characteristics of 'tension headache'. |
Student	It can affect any part of the head and it occurs at times of tension and anxiety.
Consultant	That's correct, but typically it occurs either at the top of the head at the vertex, or over the eyes in the frontal region. Do you know what kind of headache it is?
Student	It is usually a constant ache.
Consultant	It can be, but more frequently it's a feeling of pressure like 'a weight on the top of the head', or it's often described as like 'a tight band' around the head. It may last only for seconds, or for hours or even days at a time. I think we can dismiss this diagnosis as Mrs D.'s headache is nothing like this.

Now, I wonder if we can turn to the other interesting symptom mentioned by Mrs D. in relation to her vision, that it 'is going a bit funny', when she has the headache — what do you make of this? |
Student	She said she had difficulty in focusing with the headache and wasn't able to read. You can get disturbances of vision in migraine but I don't think that it is difficulty in focusing.
Consultant	What's the usual visual manifestation in migraine?
Student	You see flashing lights.
Consultant	Yes, typically they take on a zig-zag shape or, less convincing, like the outline of the battlements in a castle, so that they are called 'fortification spectra'. These visual hallucinations — because that is what they are — are also known as teichopsia. What Mrs D. describes is really blurring of vision; does this suggest anything to you when it occurs with the headache?
Student	Could it be due to raised intracranial pressure again?
Consultant	That is possible.

What about the tingling in the left leg? Is this relevant? |
| Student | I wondered about this. The fact that she has apparently had it for some |

	time would make it less important in relation to her present problem; otherwise, I would have considered it as a possible sign of cerebral involvement.
Consultant	That's a good point. We might get some help perhaps in deciding which it is by asking Mrs D. more specifically about the distribution of the tingling in the leg. Do you know what I am getting at?
Student	No, I'm sorry, I'm not quite clear.
Consultant	If Mrs D.'s tingling was due to her disc problem you would expect the tingling to be in a root distribution, for example down the lateral side of the leg if L 5 is affected. On the other hand, if the paraesthesiae have a cerebral origin you would expect the whole of the leg to be involved. Mrs D., can you tell us which part of your leg tingles?
Patient	It seems to occur over the whole of my leg and not just on one side, though when I used to have my disc problem the pain was on the outside of the leg.
Consultant	There seems to be little doubt, therefore, that Mrs D.'s tingling is not from her spine but more likely arising in the brain and this may obviously be relevant in association with the headache. What part of the brain might be involved?
Student	I would think that the sensory cortex was involved.
Consultant	And whereabouts in the brain is the sensory cortex?
Student	I think it's in the post-central gyrus.
Consultant	Top or bottom?
Student	The body image is represented upside-down in this gyrus, so tingling in the leg would point to the top of the sensory area.
Consultant	Well done. I'm glad that you remember your neurological anatomy. I've always felt that medical students had to learn a lot of unnecessary anatomy that many of them would never need to use. In the case of neurological diagnosis, however, anatomy is a very useful tool and the long hours of sweated labour learning it are well worth while! What are your views on the possible nature of Mrs D.'s brain lesion? Is there anything in the history which might give some help in deciding?
Student	The only thing I can think of is the smoking which might suggest a possible primary lesion in the lung.
Consultant	Yes, I agree that this is also something that we will have to keep in mind. Has she ever had any haemoptysis?
Student	I asked her about this and she has never noticed blood in her sputum, which is usually grey, except when she has bronchitis, when it is usually yellow or green.
Consultant	What about weight loss?
Student	I'm sorry, I should have asked Mrs D. about her weight. Mrs D., has there been any change in your weight recently.

Patient	I have lost some weight in the last few months but I put this down to being off my food. I've not really felt much like eating because of the headaches and the vomiting.
Consultant	The anorexia and the loss of weight may be relevant in relation to the diagnosis we have in mind. I think we have now got as much as we can from the history so let's try to summarize our conclusions, but before we do this, let me ask you — as the politicians say — a hypothetical question: if Mrs D. was aged 18, and not 55, and was obese — which in fact she isn't — is there any other diagnosis that you might consider to account for her headache?
Student	I don't know what you are getting at.
Consultant	I'm thinking of benign intracranial hypertension which occurs typically in obese young women, often with menstrual disturbances. Now, our conclusions from the history:

HISTORY

- Mrs D. has a past history of migraine
- she has had a recent exacerbation of her headache which is not like the migrainous headaches in the past
- the occurrence of the headaches at night and on waking suggest the likelihood of raised intracranial pressure
- the blurring of vision with the headache supports the possibility of raised intracranial pressure
- she also has hypertension which is another possible cause of the headache
- the paraesthesiae in the left leg may be due to a lesion in the right cerebral hemisphere
- the long history of smoking, accompanied by the anorexia and the loss of weight may indicate a possible primary lung lesion which might then subsequently involve the brain

Consultant	Now, I would like you to present your examination findings, and can I ask you to keep in mind the likely diagnoses we have discussed in the history and present the findings accordingly; perhaps you might, therefore, like to start with the nervous system (Figure 8.1).
Student	Mrs D. is well-orientated and not confused. I examined the cranial nerves first and the main abnormality was in the optic discs which I thought were blurred.
Consultant	You've focused down well on the problem — if you'll excuse the not very good pun — and this is obviously a very important finding. However, it might be better for your examination practice if you told us more systematically about the examination of the cranial nerves.
Student	Well, I didn't test the olfactory nerve.

Consultant	No one ever seems to these days. I think that's acceptable providing there are no symptoms relating to taste or smell.
Student	Her visual acuity seemed alright — she could see and count all my fingers.
Consultant	That's too crude a test of visual acuity. The simplest test is to ask her to read a newspaper; would you like to ask her to do that?
	The student asks Mrs D. to read the daily paper. He finds that, although she has no problem with the headlines and large print, she does have some difficulty with the small print which she says looks blurred.
Consultant	Obviously, the visual acuity is impaired and this is likely to be caused by the optic nerve swelling to which you referred earlier. Did you test the pupils?
Student	Yes, the light and accommodation reflexes were normal.
Consultant	To continue with the examination of the optic nerve, perhaps you could tell us now about the visual fields?
Student	I tested them by confrontation and couldn't find any obvious abnormality.
Consultant	Would you expect to find an abnormality in the presence of papilloedema?
Student	I don't think so.
Consultant	You do in fact get some constriction of the periphery of the fields but this would be difficult to find using confrontation and would really require accurate perimetry to pick it up. Did you see any retinal changes to go with the papilloedema?
Student	I couldn't see the retina well because the pupils were too small.
Consultant	Then you should have asked sister to dilate them for you with some tropicamide eye-drops, provided she doesn't have a history of glaucoma. Sister, would you mind dilating the pupils for us while we carry on with the other findings in the nervous system?
Student	Eye movements were full and she didn't have any diplopia or nystagmus.
Consultant	That takes care of cranial nerves 3, 4 and 6. What about the 5th cranial nerve?
Student	Facial sensation seems normal.
Consultant	Did you check conjunctival sensation?
Student	No, I forgot this.
Consultant	Reduction of the blink reflex may be the earliest sign of 5th nerve sensory involvement, so you should always test for this. What about the motor function of V?
Student	What do you mean?

Consultant	This is something which is often forgotten. The 5th cranial nerve has a motor function as well as a sensory one — what muscles does it supply?
Student	You mean the masseters.
Consultant	The motor division of the trigeminal nerve supplies all the muscles of mastication, and so that includes the pterygoids as well as the masseters. I would point out that in practice, I have rarely found motor abnormality of the trigeminal nerve of much diagnostic significance but that doesn't mean you should never check it when you examine the cranial nerves. What about Mrs D.'s 8th nerve?
Student	I checked her hearing with my wrist watch and also with whispering and it seemed normal.
Consultant	If you do get an abnormality of hearing, don't forget to do the Rinne* and the Weber† tests. How do you test the 9th (glossopharyngeal) nerve?
Student	I usually do it with the gag reflex. It was normal.
Consultant	What about cranial nerves 10, 11 and 12?
Student	Palatal movement and tongue movement were normal.
Consultant	Good. Now let's go back to the pupils which are well dilated; what can you see in the fundus?
Student	I can see swelling of the optic discs on both sides, and I can also see some haemorrhages around the discs.
Consultant	Can you tell us whether the haemorrhages are flame-shaped or like blobs?
Student	They are flame-shaped.
Consultant	Do you know what the significance of this shape is?
Student	I think it signifies that the haemorrhages are occurring in the superficial layers of the retina.
Consultant	Good. This is a typical finding in papilloedema — and incidentally in severe hypertension also — which contrasts with the rounded haemorrhages you get in the deeper layers of the retina in conditions like diabetes. Can you comment on the retinal veins?
Student	They look distended.
Consultant	Another typical finding in acute papilloedema — venous engorgement. What is the significance of these findings?
Student	They suggest raised intracranial pressure.
Consultant	That's right. What about the rest of the neurological examination?

* H.A. Rinne (1819–1868) was a German ear, nose and throat surgeon.
† F.E. Weber-Liel (1832–1891) was also a German ear, nose and throat surgeon.

Student	With respect to the motor system first, I couldn't find any muscle weakness and I thought that the deep reflexes were normal, but I wondered whether the left plantar response was upwards.
	The consultant checks the plantar responses and demonstrates quite clearly an extensor response on the left side.
Consultant	What does this indicate?
Student	There is pyramidal involvement on the left side.
Consultant	Did you confirm this with the superficial abdominal reflexes?
Student	No, I'm sorry, I always seem to forget to do this.
Consultant	A common and regrettable omission! The abdominal reflexes are lost unilaterally in pyramidal disease and can be a useful diagnostic aid when the plantar responses are in doubt. Would you like to check this in Mrs D.?
	The student finds that the superficial abdominal reflexes on the left side are absent, but he is rebuked by the consultant for trying too many times and leaving unsightly red lines on Mrs D.'s abdomen.
Consultant	Before we leave the motor system and go on to your sensory findings, I'd like to point out that you forgot to comment on muscle wasting, muscle tone and fasciculation when you started to present your findings; try to remember to do this next time. Now what about sensation?
Student	I couldn't find any abnormality to cotton wool, pin-prick, vibration or joint position; I didn't test for temperature.
Consultant	You said in the history that she had noticed some clumsiness affecting the left hand: if sensation is normal and muscle power is normal how would you account for this?
Student	It could be due to cerebellar incoordination.
Consultant	Good. Did you test for this?
Student	Yes, I did the finger–nose test and the heel–knee test and I thought they were both normal.
Consultant	I'm glad you didn't mention dysdiadochokinesis as I have the greatest difficulty pronouncing it! So how do we explain the clumsy left hand if power is normal, sensation is normal and cerebellar function is normal?
Student	I don't know.
Consultant	You have forgotten to test another important aspect of sensation — discriminatory sensation — the control of which lies in a different part of the brain to that of the primary sensation of touch, pin-prick, vibration and temperature. Do you know where this control lies?

Student	I'm sorry, I'm not sure.
Consultant	The control of discriminatory sensation is in the parietal lobe. How would you test for parietal lobe function?
Student	You would check for astereognosis.
Consultant	Yes, that is one of the important tests, the others being impaired two-point discrimination and localization of sensory stimuli and sensory inattention.
	Sister, would you please get the dividers while the student checks Mrs D.'s stereognosis.

The student gives the patient a 50p coin, a comb, a pen and a key. He finds that she correctly identifies all the items with the right hand with her eyes closed but could only clearly identify the comb with the left hand.

Consultant	What do you think of that performance?
Student	She has astereognosis in the left hand.
Consultant	Now, sister has brought the dividers and I would like you to do the two-point discrimination test. First of all, perhaps you had better remind us of the normal amount of separation which should be recognized.
Student	I'm not sure.
Consultant	It's about 0.5 cm in the finger tips, 1 cm on the palm of the hand and 2 cm on the back of the hand.

The student finds that Mrs D. needs about 2.5 cm of separation on the palm to recognize the two points and 1.5 cm on the finger tips.

Consultant	What do you deduce from all these findings?
Student	Mrs D. is likely to have a parietal lobe lesion.
Consultant	I agree. Now check for sensory inattention.
Student	I'm not quite sure how you test for this.
Consultant	The easiest way is to stroke both of her arms at the same time and see if she feels you touching both sides: alternatively, you could use 2 pins.

The student quite rightly strokes each forearm in turn to check that primary sensation is intact on each side, and then strokes both arms together when Mrs D. seems unable to feel the left side.

Consultant	This confirms parietal lobe dysfunction on the right. What do you think is the likely cause of the parietal lobe involvement?
Student	I think that she has a space-occupying lesion.
Consultant	I agree. Now, in the light of our previous discussion about the possible origin of a space-occupying lesion in the brain, what are you particularly going to look for in the rest of your examination?

Student	I will be looking for a neoplastic lesion in the lung.
Consultant	That's right, and there is another important site you would look at in a woman, isn't there?
Student	The breasts. I checked Mrs D.'s breasts and couldn't find any abnormality.
Consultant	Would you like to tell me specifically what you would be looking for in the lungs if you were thinking of a bronchial neoplasm?
Student	Any findings in the lung such as a collapse, but I couldn't find any evidence of this when I examined her.
Consultant	What other signs might you look for if you suspect a bronchial neoplasm?
Student	Finger clubbing, which she doesn't have and enlarged glands in the axilla or the neck — I couldn't find any.
Consultant	You're doing well. Any other signs, perhaps in the abdomen?
Student	You could get an enlarged liver due to metastases but again I could not find any abnormality in the abdomen.
Consultant	Do you know any other signs due to a bronchial neoplasm?
Student	I think you can sometimes get recurrent laryngeal nerve palsy leading to a hoarse voice.
Consultant	Good, this is due to involvement of the left recurrent laryngeal nerve and will be most likely to occur with a left-sided bronchial lesion — why do I say that?
Student	Because the left recurrent laryngeal nerve loops down under the aortic arch and is therefore near the left hilum.
Consultant	Well done! Your anatomy is standing you in good stead. Do you know any other nerves which might similarly be affected?
Student	I have heard of Pancoast's* syndrome which is caused by involvement of the brachial plexus.
Consultant	Good, any other nerves that could be involved?
Student	I can't think of any more.
Consultant	You can sometimes get involvement of the sympathetic chain in the neck leading to Horner's[†] syndrome. Also we mustn't forget that a non-metastatic polyneuropathy can occur. Is there anything else you want to tell us about your examination?
Student	I've already mentioned that her blood pressure was not increased, 160/90, and the rest of the cardiovascular system was normal. She also had scattered rhonchi in the lungs.

* H.K. Pancoast (1875–1939) was an American radiologist.
† J.F. Horner (1831–1886) was Professor of Ophthalmology in Zürich.

Consultant	What is the cause of this?
Student	The most likely thing is bronchitis which is probably due to her smoking.
Consultant	Well, I think this really completes the examination and as usual we will try to summarize our conclusions:

> **EXAMINATION**
>
> - Mrs D. has definite papilloedema indicating raised intracranial pressure
> - discriminatory sensation was abnormal in the left upper limb and was associated with sensory inattention on this side — this suggests a parietal lobe lesion
> - the extensor plantar response on the left, and the absent abdominal reflexes on this side suggests early pyramidal involvement also
> - we have looked for a primary neoplastic lesion in the lung which might have metastasized to the brain but found no evidence of this
> - in summary we think that the most likely diagnosis is a primary space-occupying lesion affecting the right parietal lobe, probably neoplastic

Because of the nature of the problem, the group now retires to Sister's office to discuss the relevant investigations and management.

Consultant	Shall we now get on with the investigations? What do you think we should do first?
Student	Blood count and ESR.
Consultant	That seems to be the standard response whenever I ask for investigation of any patient whatever the condition. How will this test help in diagnosing Mrs D.?
Student	It may show that she is anaemic.
Consultant	It may but that doesn't really help us much with the diagnosis, does it?
Student	The ESR may be raised and that might suggest a neoplastic condition.
Consultant	Again I agree but a raised ESR is non-specific and so doesn't take us very much further in our diagnostic quest. Try to remember what diagnoses we had in mind when we were analysing the clinical findings.
Student	I think we should do a chest X-ray.
Consultant	That's more like it! A chest X-ray should be the first test to be done in any patient suspected of having a brain tumour because it is the commonest primary site in a cerebral metastatic lesion. Here is Mrs D.'s chest X-ray — what do you think of it?
Student	I can't see any evidence of a bronchial carcinoma, but there are heavy lung markings at the lung bases.

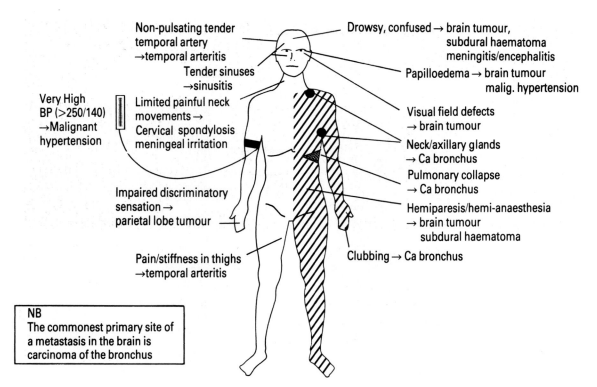

Non-pulsating tender temporal artery →temporal arteritis

Tender sinuses →sinusitis

Limited painful neck movements → Cervical spondylosis meningeal irritation

Very High BP (>250/140) →Malignant hypertension

Impaired discriminatory sensation → parietal lobe tumour

Pain/stiffness in thighs →temporal arteritis

Drowsy, confused → brain tumour, subdural haematoma meningitis/encephalitis

Papilloedema → brain tumour malig. hypertension

Visual field defects → brain tumour

Neck/axillary glands → Ca bronchus

Pulmonary collapse → Ca bronchus

Hemiparesis/hemi-anaesthesia → brain tumour subdural haematoma

Clubbing → Ca bronchus

NB
The commonest primary site of a metastasis in the brain is carcinoma of the bronchus

Figure 8.1 Possible signs of diagnostic help in a patient with headache.

Consultant	What is the explanation for that?
Student	The changes are probably due to chronic bronchitis.
Consultant	That's right. What is the next test?
Student	I think she should have a CT brain scan.
Consultant	I am very glad that you have gone to the most helpful diagnostic test of all in a patient like Mrs D.
	Here is the result of the CT scan (Figure 8.2). Are you familiar with CT scans?
Student	I've seen a few but I find it difficult sometimes to analyse unless the abnormality is very obvious.
Consultant	I think that Mrs D.'s scan shows an obvious abnormality, and on the basis of your clinical assessment you should know where in the brain to look.
Student	I can see a large rounded area with irregular shadowing in the middle of the right cerebral hemisphere.
Consultant	What do you think it is?
Student	I think it's probably a brain tumour.
Consultant	I agree. To be more specific I would say it was likely to be a parietal lobe

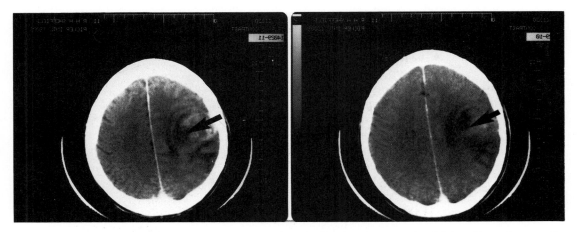

Figure 8.2   CT brain scan in Mrs D. showing a parietal lobe glioma (arrowed).

	neoplasm as we surmised in our clinical assessment. How can we get more information about its nature?
Student	We will have to do a brain biopsy.
Consultant	This is currently being arranged. If it is a cerebral neoplasm as we suspect, what treatment can we offer?
Student	It may be possible to operate and remove it.
Consultant	This will depend on whether it is primary or secondary, and if primary, the extent of the infiltration. If surgery is not possible, is there any medical treatment which will help?
Student	You could try radiotherapy or chemotherapy.
Consultant	The use of either of these treatments will depend very much on the nature and sensitivity of the neoplasm. In any case this type of treatment is only palliative. Also, we mustn't forget the value of intravenous mannitol, for acute use, and dexamethasone, in the long term, in reducing cerebral oedema which is almost invariably associated with cerebral tumours.

OUTCOME

Mrs D. had a burr biopsy. It showed a very malignant glioblastoma multiforme. Operation was not considered possible. She was treated with a combination of irradiation and carmustine to shrink the tumour, and dexamethasone to reduce the associated cerebral oedema. Her headaches improved a great deal and she was much more comfortable.

She survived for only 4 more months.

LEARNING POINTS

Main causes of headache

- migraine
- vascular disease
    - hypertension
    - temporal arteritis
    - subarachnoid haemorrhage
- space-occupying lesion
    - brain tumour
    - subdural haematoma
- local disease
    - sinusitis
    - cervical spondylosis
    - skull disease
        - Paget's disease
        - myeloma
    - eye disease
        - glaucoma
        - iridocyclitis
- tension headache

Typical features of migraine

- throbbing
- usually hemicranial (varying side)
- nausea/vomiting which often relieves the pain
- visual disturbance (teichopsia)
- triggers
    - stress
    - premenstrual week
    - alcohol (especially red wine)
    - chocolate
    - cheese

Typical features of headache due to raised intracranial pressure

- throbbing or bursting
- site
    - frontoparietal → supra-tentorial lesion
    - occipital → infra-tentorial lesion
- occurs at night and on waking
- worse on bending, straining, coughing, sneezing
- nausea/vomiting — doesn't relieve pain

Features of tension headache

- site
    - often at vertex

      frontal or occipital
      may be 'all over'
- character
      'pressure'
      'weight on the head'
      'band round the head'
      other bizarre descriptions
- lasts for hours or days
- often triggered by mental stress
- other anxiety symptoms present
      left inframammary pain
      palpitations
      can't breathe deeply enough
      tremors

Clinical features of temporal arteritis

- usually older men
- constitutional symptoms
      fever
      malaise
      loss of weight
- severe temporal headache
- tender, red, non-pulsatile temporal arteries
- optic neuritis → blindness
- muscle pains especially thighs/shoulders
- very high ESR (>100 mm/hr) — not invariable

Signs of pyramidal damage

- increased tone (spasticity)
- muscle weakness
- increased deep reflexes (often with clonus)
- absent superficial abdominal reflexes (unilateral)
- extensor plantar responses (Babinski* response)

Features of parietal lobe involvement

- impaired sensory discrimination
      point localization
      two-point separation
      stereognosis
- sensory inattention (sensory extinction)

* J.F.F. Babinski (1857–1932), of Polish origin, qualified in Paris and worked at the famous French Hospital, the Salpêtrière. Ironically, he died of Parkinson's disease.

- neglect of affected side of the body
- inability to write or calculate (lesion of dominant lobe)
- indifference to illness

Non-metastatic complications of bronchial carcinoma

- neurological
    peripheral neuropathy
    cerebellar degeneration
    'motor neurone disease' syndrome
    myasthenia gravis-like syndrome (Eaton–Lambert[*] syndrome)
    dementia (multifocal leuko-encephalopathy)
- ectopic hormones
    ADH $\rightarrow$ diabetes insipidus
    ACTH $\rightarrow$ Cushing's[†] syndrome
    gonadotrophins $\rightarrow$ gynaecomastia (males)
- thrombophlebitis migrans
- hypercalcaemia
- hypertrophic pulmonary osteoarthropathy

[*] L.M. Eaton (1905–1958) was an American neurologist at the Mayo Clinic; E.H. Lambert is a contemporary American neurophysiologist, also at the Mayo Clinic.
[†] H.W. Cushing (1869–1939) was a famous American neurosurgeon.

9

Dizziness

Student	Mr S.W. is a 68-year-old retired school caretaker who has been admitted to hospital because he had a bad fall.
	He has been dizzy on and off for about 2 years but it has been getting worse over the last few weeks. He notices the dizziness especially in the morning when he gets out of bed, but he also gets attacks of dizziness when he is up and about. He has been admitted at this time because he had a bad fall during one of these attacks of dizziness when he was out in the street and injured his shoulder and knee. He was brought to Casualty and then admitted to this ward for further investigation.
	On systematic enquiry, he said he has angina for which he takes tablets and a spray, and he also has a chronic cough which he puts down to his smoking — he smokes 15–20 cigarettes a day.
	In the past history, he has had occasional attacks of winter bronchitis for which his GP gives him antibiotics. He thinks he had high blood pressure about 10 years ago and was treated with tablets for about 18 months and then the tablets were stopped. He has had his blood pressure checked from time to time afterwards and his doctor has said it is all right.
	There was nothing relevant in the family history.
	I've already mentioned his smoking, and his drinking is very moderate — just 2 or 3 pints at weekends.
	And that's about all in the history. Shall I go on with the examination?
Consultant	No, I would prefer you to analyse the symptoms first because in most common medical problems like dizziness you are going to make the diagnosis on the basis of the history, and the examination findings are unlikely to add much to your diagnosis.
	Our problem then in Mr W. is a 2-year history of increasing dizziness, so what are your thoughts on the possible causes?
Student	It could be due to cerebrovascular insufficiency.
Consultant	I think you will have to be a bit more specific than that. What type of cerebrovascular insufficiency do you have in mind — or perhaps to put it a little more precisely, in what particular territory of the cerebral circulation do you think the problem is?

Student	I think he has vertebro-basilar insufficiency.
Consultant	This is a common problem. What part of the brain is involved?
Student	The brain stem.
Consultant	And can you think of any particular structure in the brain stem which may be affected to produce dizziness?
Student	It could be the vestibular nuclei.
Consultant	What type of dizziness would that produce?
Student	It would cause vertigo.
Consultant	What are the distinctive features of vertigo?
Student	The patient feels that the surroundings are spinning around him.
Consultant	That is what we call 'objective' vertigo. Sometimes the patient feels that he himself is spinning and not the surroundings — that is 'subjective' vertigo. 　　Was Mr W.'s dizziness true vertigo?
Student	I'm sorry I didn't go into any detail with him about the nature of his dizziness.
Consultant	Dizziness — like headache and chest pain — always needs detailed questioning on its nature to decide the cause. Regrettably, this is all too often neglected not only by students but also by housemen as well. Since the diagnosis of Mr W.'s dizziness is going to depend mainly on the history, perhaps you might like to ask him some pertinent questions about it.
Student	Mr W., can you tell us what your dizziness is like?
Patient	Sometimes the room seems to go round and round and I feel sick. I don't seem to be able to stand up when I have one of these attacks, and it was what I had when I fell down and was admitted to hospital.
Consultant	(To student) What do you make of that?
Student	It certainly sounds as if he has real vertigo.
Consultant	I agree. There are two important points he made in his answer which I think clinch the diagnosis of vertigo — the fact that he feels sick with the spinning, and also this feeling that he can't stand up — this is called 'impulsion' when the patient feels irresistably pulled or 'impelled' towards the floor. If you are in doubt about whether a patient has vertigo, 'impulsion' is an important confirmatory symptom. 　　You may have also noticed in Mr W.'s answer that he said he has vertigo only 'sometimes'. This suggests he may have other types of dizziness as well on other occasions. Would you like to ask him about this?
Student	Mr W., apart from these attacks of spinning, do you get any other sort of dizziness where the room doesn't go round — any feelings of faintness or light-headedness perhaps?

Patient	Yes, I do when I get out of bed in the morning. The room doesn't go round but I feel light-headed and unsteady, and I have to sit down on the bed again for a few minutes before it passes off.
Consultant	(To student) What are your comments on this?
Student	I think this sounds like cerebrovascular insufficiency.
Consultant	I would agree. It would appear therefore that Mr W. has two kinds of dizziness — the attacks of vertigo and the cerebrovascular insufficiency. I think we should consider each in turn, so would you like to start by telling us whether you think that Mr W.'s vertigo is arising centrally in the brain stem or peripherally from the ear?
Student	I think that the best way of deciding this would be by audiometry.
Consultant	That may be so, but don't you think we might be able to decide about the vertigo by using our own ears rather than Mr W.'s?
Student	I'm not sure what you are getting at.
Consultant	What I mean is that we can ask Mr W. some appropriate questions and then decide about the origin of his vertigo by listening to his answers with our ears. What do you think the relevant questions might be?
Student	We could ask him whether he has had any chronic ear infection.
Consultant	Yes, that would be a good start. Go ahead.
Student	Mr W., have you had any discharge from your ears in the past?
Patient	No, but I have had wax which my doctor has had to wash out a few times.
Student	He doesn't seem to have had chronic ear disease.
Consultant	Isn't there anything else you could ask him about his ears which might be relevant?
Student	We should find out whether he has tinnitus.
Consultant	Yes, that's a very important point, but before we come to this there is another question you should ask which would be just as important. If I were to give you a clue, perhaps I would suggest that you might already have asked him the question and had no reply.
Student	I'm not clear what you mean.
Consultant	I'm sorry, perhaps I'm being too subtle. (To patient) Mr W., can you tell us what your hearing is like?
Patient	I have been going a bit deaf. That's why my doctor has been washing my ears out, but it doesn't seem to have made much difference to my hearing.
Consultant	Now, if you like you can go back to the tinnitus and ask Mr W. about this.
Student	(To patient) Do you get any noises in your ears?

Patient	Yes, I do, I get a lot of ringing in my ears, especially in my left ear.
Consultant	Mr W., have you noticed whether you are deaf in both ears or on just one side?
Patient	I think it's worse in my right ear; that's also the side where I get most of the noises in my ear.
Consultant	(To student) Now, you should ask Mr W. an important supplementary question about the tinnitus which would help us a lot in deciding the cause of the vertigo.
Student	I'm sorry, I don't know which question you mean.
Consultant	Mr W., have you noticed whether the ringing in your ears is worse at any particular time?
Patient	I'll tell you when it always seems louder — it's during the bad attacks of dizziness.
Consultant	Thank you, Mr W., that is very helpful information for us. (To student) It now appears that Mr W. has a triad of symptoms — a hearing defect, attacks of vertigo, and tinnitus, which tends to get worse during the attack of vertigo. What do you think this triad of symptoms suggests?
Student	Ménière's* disease.
Consultant	Good. Although Ménière's disease is probably the commonest peripheral cause of vertigo, there are several others which we should mention.
Student	We have already referred to chronic otitis media.
Consultant	Yes, this is an important cause of involvement of the labyrinth in the inner ear. We should also mention benign positional vertigo which is worse in bed, especially on changing position, and we mustn't forget the side-effect of drugs — which drugs?
Student	Anti-convulsants used in epilepsy.
Consultant	Which ones do you have in mind?
Student	Can't all of them do it?
Consultant	No, the drug most frequently involved is phenytoin, and the other anti-convulsant which I have seen produce vertigo sometimes is primidone. Do you know any other drugs producing vertigo?
Student	Salicylates can do it.
Consultant	That's right, and they can also cause tinnitus. What about antibiotics?
Student	Streptomycin can cause vertigo.

* Prosper Ménière (1799–1862) was a French ENT surgeon who wrote his account of recurrent labyrinthine vertigo in 1861. He was a friend of Balzac and Victor Hugo.

Consultant	And deafness. The other antibiotic is gentamicin. Another drug causing vertigo is quinine, especially if taken in excess. 　　Can you think of any other peripheral cause of vertigo not involving the labyrinth?
Student	No, I'm sorry.
Consultant	You mustn't forget an acoustic neuroma; in this case the vertigo would be persistent and not intermittent as in Mr W.'s case. 　　Perhaps you can tell us now about some central causes of vertigo, by which we mean causes in the brain?
Student	It can occur in demyelinating disease.
Consultant	Yes, that is a common cause, though again the vertigo would tend to be more constant. 　　Any other causes in the brain?
Student	We mentioned vertebro-basilar ischaemia before.
Consultant	Can you get tinnitus with this?
Student	I don't think so.
Consultant	In theory it could occur if the cochlear nucleus was affected in the brain stem, but in practice it is very rare. 　　Any other central causes?
Student	I can't think of any.
Consultant	A space-occupying lesion in the posterior fossa can cause vertigo, and it can also be a manifestation of temporal lobe epilepsy. 　　Now, I would like to turn our attention to Mr W.'s other type of dizziness — when he gets out of bed. What do you think this is caused by?
Student	It is probably due to postural hypotension causing vertebro-basilar insufficiency.
Consultant	Is there any reason why he should have postural hypotension?
Student	I don't think so. He isn't having any treatment for hypertension which is the usual cause.
Consultant	Do you think he might be having any other treatment which could be responsible?
Student	The only other treatment he is having is for his angina.
Consultant	And what treatment is that?
Student	He didn't know what the tablets were called.
Consultant	Can anti-anginal treatment cause postural hypotension?
Student	It can do, because some of the drugs used for angina can also lower the blood pressure.
Consultant	Which drugs do you mean?
Student	Well, nitrates and calcium-antagonists.

Consultant	In fact, all three major drugs used in angina can lower blood pressure — nitrates, beta-blockers and calcium antagonists, though it is only nitrates and calcium antagonists which are likely to produce postural hypotension, because they are both specific vasodilators. Which do you think are more likely to lower the blood pressure — nitrates or calcium antagonists?
Student	Nitrates, I think.
Consultant	Wrong this time. The primary vasodilating effects of nitrates are on the veins and less so on the arteries. On the other hand, calcium antagonists dilate the arteries only, so are more likely to cause a postural drop in blood pressure. (To patient) Mr W., are you having orange capsules for your angina?
Patient	That's right, I take one capsule 3 times a day.
Consultant	(To student) Do you know what these are.
Student	I'm sorry I don't.
Consultant	It's always useful to know what your patient's tablets or capsules look like. To go even further, one of my previous chiefs, now sadly dead, used to require his juniors not only to identify the tablets but actually to try them also. It is not a practice I follow — perhaps too many tablets in the past has put me off, but it was certainly effective in keeping our drug prescribing within reasonable bounds! To get back to Mr W.'s capsules, these are likely to be nifedipine (Adalat), which is a calcium antagonist and may well be contributing to the postural hypotension. Are there any other common contributory factors you can think of in patients with vertebro-basilar insufficiency?
Student	Cervical spondylosis is an important factor.
Consultant	And do you think Mr W. has cervical spondylosis?
Student	I didn't ask him specifically about his neck.
Consultant	Well, I think you should.
Student	Mr W., do you have any trouble with your neck?
Patient	I do get aching at the back of my neck sometimes — my doctor said it was due to 'fibrositis'.
Consultant	(To student) Do you think that Mr W.'s pain is due to cervical spondylosis or 'fibrositis'.
Student	Probably spondylosis.
Consultant	Is there any other question you could ask which would tell you more definitely whether Mr W. had cervical spondylosis?
Student	I'm not sure.
Consultant	Mr W., do you ever feel a crunching or creaking sensation in your neck when you move your head?

Patient	Yes, I have noticed a crunching especially when it's very quiet and I slowly turn my head from side to side.
Consultant	This indicates that Mr W. does have cervical spondylosis. How would you decide whether this is a significant factor in causing his dizziness?
Student	A neck X-ray would show us.
Consultant	It might well confirm the cervical spondylosis but it still wouldn't help in deciding how much it was contributing to the dizziness. In any case, we are still considering the history and not investigations.
Student	I'm not sure what else will help in the history.
Consultant	(To patient) Mr W., have you ever noticed whether turning your head or looking up has any effect on the dizziness?
Patient	If I turn my head quickly to the side, or if I look up to the ceiling, I sometimes feel dizzy and light-headed for a few seconds.
Consultant	(To student) It is apparent that the cervical spondylosis is relevant to his dizziness. 　　What do you think the mechanism is?
Student	I think it's due to pressure on the vertebral arteries by the arthritic neck joints because the arteries are close to the joints.
Consultant	That's right. If Mr W. were to tell us that his dizziness occurred mainly on physical exertion, especially when he was using his arms, would that suggest anything else to you?
Student	I don't think so.
Consultant	Have you heard of the 'subclavian steal syndrome'?
Student	I've heard of it, but I've never been very clear as to how it works.
Consultant	It is due to atheromatous obstruction of the subclavian artery proximal to the origin of the vertebral artery. During vigorous exertion using the affected arm, blood is diverted from the basilar system by retrograde flow through the vertebral artery to the subclavian artery distal to the obstruction — this leads to basilar ischaemia and dizziness.
Student	That's the first time I have ever really understood the mechanism.
Consultant	Now, I would like to go back to Mr W.'s fall when he injured his knee and his shoulder. He said that he fell during one of his severe attacks of vertigo. If he had told us that he fell without any preceding dizziness, would that suggest any alternative cause to you?
Student	I wouldn't really know what the cause would be.
Consultant	Have you heard of 'drop attacks'?
Student	Yes, I think they can occur in cerebrovascular insufficiency.
Consultant	Not in general cerebrovascular insufficiency but only with ischaemia of the brain stem. The patient usually has no warning, drops suddenly, recovers in a few seconds and feels quite well afterwards.

Now, I think we've discussed Mr W.'s main symptoms so perhaps we can try to summarize our conclusions:

HISTORY

- Mr W. has two types of dizziness — attacks of true vertigo and vertebro-basilar insufficiency
- the association of deafness and tinnitus with the vertigo indicates that the likely cause is Ménière's disease
- Mr W.'s neck pain and 'crunching' on neck movement indicates that he has cervical spondylosis
- the exacerbation of Mr W.'s light-headedness with neck movement shows that the cervical spondylosis is contributing to his vertebrobasilar insufficiency
- it is likely that the peripheral vasodilating action of the nifedipine, which he is taking for his angina, is helping to cause his postural dizziness

Consultant	Now, I would like you to present your examination findings and remember that our main concern is with Mr W.'s dizziness — this means that your presentation is problem-orientated and based on the diagnoses we have discussed in the history (Figure 9.1).
Student	Mr W. is lying comfortably in bed.
Consultant	A traditional start but could you try to be more specific and less routine.
Student	I'll tell you about his cardio-vascular system first because we think one of his problems is cerebrovascular insufficiency.
Consultant	On that basis I would have thought that the nervous system would be a more appropriate start. However, carry on!
Student	His pulse was irregularly-irregular.
Consultant	Due to what?
Student	It could be due to ectopic beats or it could be due to atrial fibrillation.
Consultant	In practice, an irregularly-irregular pulse is very rarely due to multiple ectopic beats and much more likely to be due to atrial fibrillation.
Student	His pulse rate was 96/min, the blood pressure was 170/100, I couldn't feel the apex beat and I thought the heart sounds were normal with no murmurs.
Consultant	How would you interpret these findings?
Student	He is likely to have atrial fibrillation and he has mild hypertension.
Consultant	Are they relevant to Mr W.'s dizziness?
Student	They could be. The hypertension could lead to the dizziness.
Consultant	I'm glad you said 'lead to' and not 'cause'. It is a widespread miscon-

ception that high blood pressure causes dizziness as one of the earliest symtoms. Dizziness in hypertension is due to associated cerebrovascular disease as a result of the cerebral arteriosclerosis which develops in long-standing hypertension and is not therefore a specific symptom of hypertension itself. In fact there are very few symptoms directly attributable to hypertension, perhaps epistaxis and also headache in severe hypertension, are the only two symptoms which I would regard as likely to be due directly to hypertension.

Mr W.'s hypertension may therefore be relevant to his dizziness by leading to vertebro-basilar arteriosclerosis and ischaemia.

Did you check his standing blood pressure?

Student	No, I'm sorry I forgot to do this.
Consultant	Do you think it is important?
Student	Yes, it is because he was complaining of feeling dizzy when he gets out of bed and we thought this was likely to be due to postural hypotension. I'll check it now.

The student finds a lying blood pressure of 170/100 and a standing blood pressure of 130/90.

Student	He does have a postural fall.
Consultant	This is likely to be relevant to the complaint of postural dizziness and is presumably attributable to the treatment with nifedipine. Did you find any evidence of arteriosclerosis?
Student	I thought his foot pulses were poor.
Consultant	Anything else?
Student	The fundal arteries look narrowed and irregular.
Consultant	Good. The fundi are probably the best guide of all to arteriosclerosis since it is the only part of the body where you can actually see the arteries. The other useful indicator of arteriosclerosis is a tortuous brachial artery which is called a locomotor brachial artery. Has Mr W. got a locomotor brachial artery?
Student	I didn't look specifically.

The student looks at the patient's arm — there is a well-marked tortuous, pulsating brachial artery.

Consultant	There is little doubt that Mr W. has significant arteriosclerosis. Another sign of arteriosclerosis that you would look for is a murmur over the carotid arteries in the neck, which might be very relevant in Mr W.'s case because we think he has vertebro-basilar insufficiency. Does he have a murmur over his carotid arteries?

Student	I'm afraid that I didn't listen.
Consultant	Unfortunately, listening over the carotid arteries is often forgotten. You would be wise to incorporate it as a routine part of your examination of the cardio-vascular system if not in the nervous system. I think you had better listen now to Mr W.'s carotid arteries.

The student finds that Mr W. does have a rough systolic murmur over the right carotid artery.

Consultant	What do you think that indicates?
Student	It confirms that he has narrowing of the carotid artery due to atherosclerosis.
Consultant	If there is atherosclerosis of the carotid arteries then it is likely that the cerebral and vertebro-basilar arteries are similarly affected. Incidentally, if you do hear a murmur over the carotid artery you should always confirm that it is not simply conducted up from a diseased aortic valve. The other signs to look for in arteriosclerosis are a murmur over the abdominal aorta — which Mr W. does not have — and premature arcus senilis in a young man, especially if there is xanthelasma also. You said earlier that Mr W. is likely to have atrial fibrillation and you gave us his pulse rate of 96/min. Do you think that the pulse rate is a reliable indication of heart rate in atrial fibrillation?
Student	I think so; it tells us if the heart is going too fast.
Consultant	It is not in fact a reliable guide, is it, because some of the heart beats may not come through to the wrist if the beat is very premature with a poor stroke volume, which is often the case in uncontrolled atrial fibrillation. Therefore you should always count the apex rate by auscultation when you find atrial fibrillation; this is particularly important when you are assessing efficacy of control with digoxin treatment. What do you think is the likely cause of Mr W.'s atrial fibrillation?
Student	Most likely it is his underlying coronary disease.
Consultant	I agree, as Mr W. has angina. Even in the absence of angina I think that coronary artery disease is one of the commonest causes of otherwise unexplained — sometimes called 'lone' — atrial fibrillation. Can you tell us any other causes of atrial fibrillation?
Student	You can get it in rheumatic heart disease.
Consultant	Yes, especially in mitral stenosis. What else?
Student	Thyrotoxicosis.
Consultant	Any other causes?
Student	I can't think of any others.
Consultant	It occurs often, in my experience, in hypertension but I think this could

be due to associated, and perhaps clinically undetected, coronary artery disease. Other causes include infective myocarditis, primary and secondary cardiomyopathy, bronchial carcinoma infiltrating the atrium and atrial septal defect — all these causes are rare.

Now, to return to the examination, what do you want to tell us about next?

Student   We've dealt with the cardiovascular system so shall I go on to the respiratory system?

Consultant   Since his main problem is his dizziness I would have thought that the more relevant system to take next should be the nervous system, unless it was thought that the cause of the dizziness was in the respiratory system — we'll come back to this point later.

What did you look for when you examined the nervous system?

Student   I looked for focal signs, especially in the cranial nerves because of the likelihood of brain-stem ischaemia.

Consultant   Which cranial nerves do you think are likely to be involved in brain-stem ischaemia?

Student   I would think that it is the lower cranial nerves, say from the 8th downwards.

Consultant   If the midbrain and upper pons are involved in the ischaemia then it is likely to affect the 3rd, 4th and 6th cranial nerves and this would cause . . . ?

Student   Double vision.

Consultant   That's right. If the ischaemia affected the lower pons and medulla you might get involvement of the 8th cranial nerve leading to vertigo or sometimes the 10th nerve which might cause some dysarthria.

Do you think that the 5th and the 7th nerves could be relevant in any way to Mr W.'s problems?

Student   I can't think of any connection unless they were involved in the ischaemia.

Consultant   This doesn't happen very often in brain-stem ischaemia. I wondered whether you might see any relevance particularly to Mr W.'s vertigo.

Student   I'm sorry, I don't.

Consultant   I was thinking of an acoustic neuroma. You will, I am sure, remember that the 8th nerve is close to both the 7th nerve and the 5th nerve in the brain stem. You might find a loss of corneal sensation which is your only clinical clue to the possibility of an acoustic neuroma on examination.

Now, tell us your cranial nerve findings.

Student   I couldn't find any abnormality in the optic nerve — his vision was all right and the optic discs looked normal; his external ocular movements were normal; sensation was normal over the face and the movements were normal. The only abnormality was his hearing which was reduced in the right ear. Palatal and tongue movements were normal.

Consultant	That was a good account of your examination of the cranial nerves, and you should always specify the individual nerves as you have done. I'd like to pick you up on the hearing problem. Did you look into his ears with an auroscope?
Student	I'm sorry, I didn't.
Consultant	This is something you must always do in a patient with a hearing problem. If you're very lucky you will find the ear blocked with wax and you can then perform a 'miraculous' cure with ear syringing. The other important reason is to look for evidence of chronic middle ear infection in the eardrum. Can you tell us whether Mr W. has conduction deafness or nerve deafness?
Student	I don't think so.
Consultant	Did you not do the Weber* and Rinne[†] tests?
Student	No, I'm sorry I didn't remember to do them, but I will do them now.

The student does the tests: the Weber test is referred to the left ear, and the Rinne test shows that bone conduction is better than air conduction in the right ear but a normal response is present in the left ear.

Consultant	What do these results mean?
Student	He has nerve deafness affecting the right ear.
Consultant	This would be consistent with the diagnosis of Ménière's disease. We have already discussed the function of the other cranial nerves — did you find any abnormality?
Student	No, the other cranial nerves were normal.
Consultant	The only other sign that you might find sometimes in Ménière's disease is nystagmus, but you would be more likely to find this if you examined the patient during an acute attack. If you had found nystagmus, would you know how to distinguish brain-stem nystagmus from labyrinthine nystagmus, because brain-stem ischaemia can also lead to nystagmus?
Student	I have always found difficulty in deciding the origin of nystagmus.
Consultant	The simplest method is to note whether the nystagmus increases when the patient looks to one side: if it increases when looking away from the side where you suspect the lesion then it is labyrinthine in origin; on

* F.E. Weber-Liel (1832–1891) was a German ENT specialist. (He is not to be confused with Sir H.D. Weber (1823–1918) who was a physician at Guy's Hospital and described Weber's syndrome due to a lesion in the midbrain affecting eye movements on the same side and producing hemiplegia on the other side.)
[†] H.A. Rinne (1819–1868) was also a German ENT surgeon.

the other hand, if the nystagmus is due to involvement of a cerebellar tract in the brain-stem then it will increase looking towards the side of the lesion.

There are two other helpful findings in brain-stem nystagmus which don't occur with labyrinthine nystagmus — do you know what they are?

Student	Can brain-stem nystagmus be vertical?
Consultant	Yes, that is one of the distinctive findings — do you know the other?
Student	I'm sorry I don't know.
Consultant	Have you heard of ataxic nystagmus?
Student	Yes, but I'm not sure what it means.
Consultant	It means that the nystagmus is always more marked in the abducting eye. Ataxic nystagmus is a very distinctive sign in brain-stem involvement by a demyelinating disorder. Now, what about the rest of the nervous system — did you find any other abnormality?
Student	I couldn't find any abnormality of the motor system but I thought that there might be slight impairment of vibration sense at the ankles.
Consultant	Which tracts in the spinal cord carry vibration?
Student	The posterior columns.
Consultant	And what other signs would you expect to find if the posterior columns were affected?
Student	You get loss of joint position sense, but I checked this in Mr W. and it was normal.
Consultant	Then it is very unlikely that the loss of vibration sense is clinically significant; it's not uncommon to find slight impairment of vibration sense in elderly patients without any other neurological signs and it is regarded as of no clinical significance. Now, I think you should complete your examination by telling us about the respiratory and alimentary systems.
Student	When I examined his lungs I thought he was a bit wheezy.
Consultant	Not a very scientific presentation of your lung findings, is it but certainly terse and to the point! If you are doing your finals I would strongly recommend that you follow the conventional *inspection, palpation, percussion and auscultation* when discussing lung findings. However, I won't ask you to do this just now, but I will ask you to tell us what you think is causing the *rhonchi* — not 'wheezes', please!
Student	I think it is due to chronic bronchitis.
Consultant	Yes, that is the obvious cause. Do you know any specific relationship between chronic bronchitis and dizziness?
Student	I don't think so.
Consultant	Have you heard of 'cough epilepsy'?

Student	Yes, it's due to a prolonged bout of coughing causing an epileptic fit.
Consultant	That's right, but you may not always get a fit — it may just cause dizziness. The mechanism is analogous to an interesting physiological manoeuvre which you probably carried out in your pre-clinical years when you were doing your practical physiology — do you know to what I'm referring?
Student	You mean the Valsalva* manoeuvre?
Consultant	That's right. Would you like to explain the physiology of the manoeuvre to us?
Student	Not really, but I think it leads to a fall in cardiac output which can then cause unconsciousness.
Consultant	That's not bad! The increase in intrathoracic pressure with the straining of the manoeuvre prevents adequate venous return to the heart which then leads to the fall in cardiac output — this can be severe enough in a prolonged bout of coughing to cause syncope. When the strain is released you get a reflex overshoot of the blood pressure, mediated by the sympathetic system, which is accompanied by a compensatory bradycardia. This test has a lot of applications, one of which is a test of the integrity of the sympathetic nervous system. Did you examine his neck in view of the possibility of cervical spondylosis?
Student	Yes, I did and I found that Mr W. has severely limited movement especially when I tried to flex his neck laterally.
Consultant	That is always the most sensitive movement to pick up cervical spondylosis, so you have confirmed this diagnosis. What about his knee and shoulder — you said he injured both when he fell?
Student	I checked his shoulder which is bruised as you can see. His movements were a little painful but I didn't think there was any real damage. I couldn't find anything much wrong with his knee either.
Consultant	Finally, what about the alimentary system — was there anything of interest you want to tell us about?
Student	No, I don't think so. I thought that the mouth, throat and abdomen were all normal. Well, at this stage we should summarize our findings and their significance. Now, I would like to turn our attention to investigation of Mr W.'s problems. How should we start?
Student	We could start with an X-ray of his neck.

* A.M. Valsalva (1666–1723) was Professor of Anatomy at Bologna and described his famous manoeuvre in a book he published in 1704 on the ear — he used the manoeuvre as a means of insufflating the Eustachian tube.

EXAMINATION

- the only abnormal neurological finding was deafness in the right ear
- the Weber and the Rinne tests indicated that the deafness was due to involvement of the auditory nerve and not a conduction-type deafness. This is consistent with the diagnosis of Ménière's disease
- we have confirmed postural hypotension; the nifedipine treatment, for his angina, may be a contributory factor here
- he has evidence of arteriosclerosis in the brachial artery and foot arteries as well as in the fundal arterioles
- he has a systolic murmur over the right carotid artery in the neck indicating carotid atheroma
- we have confirmed cervical spondylosis which is also likely to be aggravating the vertebro-basilar insufficiency
- he has atrial fibrillation probably due to the coronary disease
- he has evidence of chronic bronchitis which is likely to be due to his heavy smoking

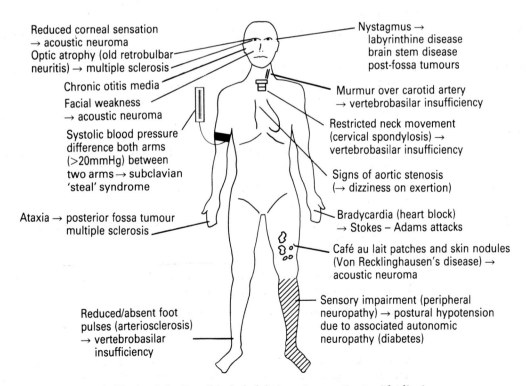

Reduced corneal sensation → acoustic neuroma
Optic atrophy (old retrobulbar neuritis) → multiple sclerosis
Chronic otitis media
Facial weakness → acoustic neuroma
Systolic blood pressure difference both arms (>20mmHg) between two arms → subclavian 'steal' syndrome
Ataxia → posterior fossa tumour multiple sclerosis
Reduced/absent foot pulses (arteriosclerosis) → vertebrobasilar insufficiency

Nystagmus → labyrinthine disease brain stem disease post-fossa tumours
Murmur over carotid artery → vertebrobasilar insufficiency
Restricted neck movement (cervical spondylosis) → vertebrobasilar insufficiency
Signs of aortic stenosis (→ dizziness on exertion)
Bradycardia (heart block) → Stokes – Adams attacks
Café au lait patches and skin nodules (Von Recklinghausen's disease) → acoustic neuroma
Sensory impairment (peripheral neuropathy) → postural hypotension due to associated autonomic neuropathy (diabetes)

Figure 9.1 Possible helpful signs in a patient with dizziness.

Consultant	And what would you look for in this X-ray?
Student	It should show us whether he has cervical spondylosis.
Consultant	Haven't you already shown that in your clinical assessment?
Student	I suppose we have, but the X-ray would show us how severe it is.
Consultant	It might, but remember you can find quite severe degenerative changes in the cervical spine in otherwise asymptomatic patients — in fact most patients over 60 have some degree of cervical spondylosis in their neck X-ray.

If you do find cervical spondylosis on X-ray, the important question to decide is whether it is clinically significant. This can only be done from the history, to determine whether it is producing any relevant symptoms, and from the examination by showing that neck movement is causing pain or dizziness.

There is one finding, however, in the neck X-ray which may be of clinical significance and you might well see it in a patient like Mr W. — do you know what I have in mind? |
| *Student* | I'm sorry, I don't know. |
| *Consultant* | You may see calcification in the carotid artery in the neck: if the patient is also getting transient ischaemic attacks, this would have implications for treatment — it would suggest the desirability of aspirin or anti-coagulants to prevent thrombus developing in the diseased carotid artery with the risk of subsequent cerebral emboli.

Here is Mr W.'s cervical spine X-ray (Figure 9.2). Would you like to give us your views on it? |
Student	There is no doubt about the cervical spondylosis.
Consultant	What about this linear shadow here?
Student	Is that a calcified carotid artery?
Consultant	That's right, and it fits in with your finding of a carotid murmur over the carotid artery. What does it mean?
Student	If confirms that Mr W. has carotid atheroma.
Consultant	That's right and is obviously an important contributory factor in producing Mr W.'s cerebrovascular insufficiency.

Do we need any other tests? |
| *Student* | I think we should confirm the Ménière's disease by audiometry. |
| *Consultant* | Audiometry would show low frequency loss and loudness recruitment in Ménière's disease but remember that the diagnosis of Ménière's disease is primarily a clinical one and based on the triad of symptoms — vertigo, deafness and tinnitus.

If we were thinking of an acoustic neuroma rather than Ménière's disease, what other tests would we need to do? |
| *Student* | We could X-ray the skull. |

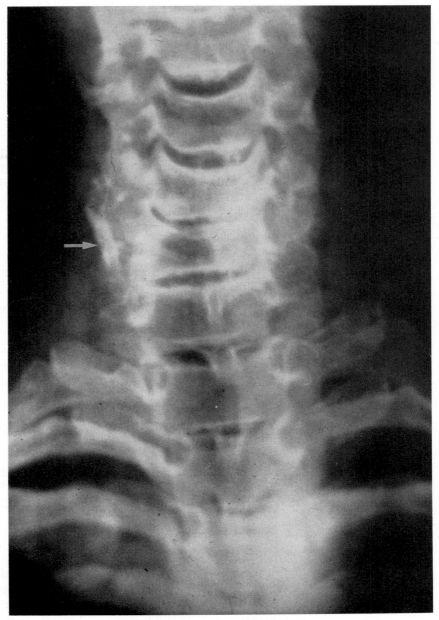

Figure 9.2 X-ray of the cervical spine showing cervical spondylosis and calcification of the carotid arteries in the neck (arrowed).

Consultant	What might we find?
Student	You might see erosion of the internal auditory meatus.
Consultant	That's very good. What would be the best test to confirm the diagnosis?
Student	I'm not sure.
Consultant	A CT scan should show you the neuroma. Any other tests for Mr W.?
Student	He should have an ECG to confirm the atrial fibrillation.

Consultant	I agree that we should have an ECG but I doubt if it will help us very much in the management of the atrial fibrillation. What would be more helpful is that it will show us whether the hypertension has had any effect on Mr W.'s heart, which is of prognostic significance.
	    Mr W.'s ECG confirmed the atrial fibrillation but didn't show any left ventricular hypertrophy.
	    Do you want any other tests?

Student	I'd like a chest X-ray.
Consultant	For what purpose?
Student	To see if he has any cardiac enlargement.
Consultant	That would also be of prognostic significance. Has the chest X-ray any other value in a patient with vertigo?
Student	It might show a bronchial neoplasm with subsequent cerebral involvement.
Consultant	This is a possibility, but in my experience it is very rare for metastatic disease of the brain to present primarily with vertigo. Do you want any other tests?
Student	We could do the blood urea and electrolytes because he is hypertensive and it will show us whether the hypertension has damaged his kidneys.
Consultant	That's a reasonable suggestion, with one proviso — you don't need the electrolytes to assess renal function — the blood urea and serum creatinine will tell you whether renal failure is present. Try to restrict your requests to what you really want to know, and avoid blanket terms like 'urea and electrolytes'. Have you finished your tests now?
Student	I can't think of any more.
Consultant	I'm inclined to agree — I think we have mentioned all the relevant tests for Mr W. If we had any real doubt that Mr W.'s neurological symptoms were due to a combination of Ménière's disease and cerebrovascular insufficiency — which we don't — then perhaps we would consider a CT scan of the brain, though it is not particularly good at showing specific lesions in the brain-stem.

OUTCOME

The diagnosis of Ménière's disease was confirmed by an ENT surgeon clinically and with audiometry. He thought it would be worth trying gromets in the tympanic membrane and this resulted in considerable improvement, with no further attacks over an 18-month follow-up period.

The treatment of Mr W.'s angina was changed from nifedipine to isosorbide mononitrate to avoid the postural hypotension. He was given a plastic collar to restrict neck movement and so reduce the tendency to vertebro-basilar insufficiency. With these two measures Mr W.'s light-headedness also improved and he was very grateful.

As far as the mild hypertension was concerned it was decided not to treat this with hypotensive drugs because of Mr W.'s susceptibility to cerebrovascular insufficiency.

Finally, he was advised to take aspirin 75 mg daily long term in view of the carotid disease in the neck to reduce the risk of transient ischaemic attacks — the aspirin will help to prevent platelet-induced thrombosis in the atheromatous carotid artery.

LEARNING POINTS

Diagnostic triad in labyrinthine disease

- vertigo
- tinnitus
- deafness

Causes of vertigo

- vertebro-basilar ischaemia
- Ménière's disease
- chronic middle ear disease
- vestibular neuronitis (acute labyrinthitis)
- acoustic neuroma
- benign positional vertigo
- drugs
    salicylates
    phenytoin
    quinine
    antibiotics
       streptomycin
       gentamicin

Weber and Rinne tests in middle ear and inner ear disease

	Weber test	*Rinne test*
Middle ear disease (conduction deafness)	louder on affected side	bone > air on affected side
Inner ear disease (nerve deafness)	louder on normal side	air > bone but both reduced

Differentiation between labyrinthine and central nystagmus

Labyrinthine	*Central*
Horizontal/rotatory	horizontal/vertical
Increases looking away from affected side	increases looking towards affected side (cerebellar)
Conjugate (both eyes similar)	ataxic (worse in abducting eye)

Treatment of Ménière's disease

- medical
    antihistamines e.g. betahistine (Serc)
    salt and water restriction
    diuretics

- surgical
    insertion of gromets
    endolymphatic drainage
    subarachnoid shunt
    section of vestibular nerve
    labyrinthectomy

Signs of arteriosclerosis

- premature arcus senilis
- xanthelasma
- thickened radial artery
- locomotor brachialis
- reduced/absent foot pulses
- fundal arteriosclerosis
- systolic murmur over the abdominal aorta
- systolic murmur over the carotid artery

Risk factors in atheroma

- major
    cigarette smoking
    hypertension
    high blood cholesterol
- minor
    family history of *premature* arterial disease
    diabetes
    obesity
    contraceptive pill (especially in smokers)
    'soft' water
    ? stress
    ? physical inactivity
    ? type A personality

Clinical manifestations of transient ischaemic attacks

- vision
    loss of vision in one eye
    double vision
    hemi-anopia
- speech
    dysarthria
    dysphasia
- sensory
    facial paraesthesiae (especially circumoral)
    paraesthesiae in the limbs

- motor
    weakness in face
    weakness in the limbs
- transient amnesia

Clinical manifestations of vertebro-basilar insufficiency

- vertigo
- light-headedness
- loss of vision in both eyes
- drop attacks
- unsteadiness (ataxia)

Features of the subclavian 'steal' syndrome

- dizziness on exercising the affected arm
- unequal radial pulses
- systolic blood pressure 20+ mmHg less in affected arm
- possible systolic murmur over supra-clavicular fossa

Drugs causing postural hypotension

- peripheral vasodilators
    hydralazine
    prazosin
    angiotensin converting enzyme inhibitors (captopril, enalapril)
- adrenergic-blockers
    guanethidine
    debrisoquine
- anti-anginal
    calcium antagonists (nifedipine; verapamil)
    nitrates (sorbide nitrate)

10

Difficulty in walking

Student	Mr T.M. is a 33-year-old welder. He was referred to you for investigation of difficulty in walking. For the last month or so he has noticed stiffness in his legs when he is walking, usually after a distance of about two or three miles on the flat. He describes his legs as feeling 'wooden', and although he hasn't noticed any particular weakness in the legs he does say that sometimes the left foot seems to drag and the toe catches in the ground. He hasn't had any pain in the legs, particularly when he has been walking, but he has noticed that his legs have been feeling heavy at times. He can't remember having had any previous trouble with the legs. The other symptom he complains of over the last few weeks is some unsteadiness and a tendency to lose his balance, especially when he walks upstairs.

I asked him whether he had any problems with his eyesight in the past; although he denies any episodes of double vision he has noticed blurring of vision occasionally. There was nothing else relevant on direct enquiry: he does not suffer with headache and has never had any fits, he has had no serious illnesses in the past that he knows of. In fact he has always led a very active life, including such things as playing football regularly and weight training — he only stopped when his legs became stiff and difficult to move.

There was nothing of significance in the family history. He smokes about 20 cigarettes a day and drinks about 4 to 5 pints of beer at the weekend. He is not taking any drug treatment at present.

Consultant	I'd like you to analyse the history for us and tell us what these symptoms suggest to you in the way of possible diagnoses.
Student	My first thoughts were that it sounds as if he has a problem with spasticity in his legs.
Consultant	Yes, I would agree that is the first point to make. His description of 'wooden' legs is very unusual and I certainly have not heard it before; it is very suggestive of spastic legs. Now I think you said that the stiffness came on after about 2 or 3 miles, and you also mentioned that there was no pain in the legs, when he was walking — did you have any other diagnosis in mind when you made this comment?

Student	I did just wonder about intermittent claudication in view of the relationship of the stiffness of the legs to the walking.
Consultant	You were quite right to think of that as sometimes a patient with claudication will complain of stiffness or heaviness of the legs rather than pain. Is there any other reason for you to suspect that he might be a candidate for peripheral vascular disease which might lead to claudication?
Student	He is a heavy smoker.
Consultant	I wouldn't call it heavy but I would agree that it may well be a factor in causing atherosclerosis in Mr M. and I'm sure that you will be telling us more about the presence or otherwise of arteriosclerosis in Mr M. when you go over your examination findings with us later. Apart from intermittent claudication is there any other condition you should keep in mind if a patient gets neurological symptoms during walking?
Student	Do you mean other than actual neurological disease?
Consultant	Yes, apart from a neurological disorder.
Student	I can't think of any other condition.
Consultant	Spinal stenosis is what I had in mind. Do you know what this is?
Student	I've heard of it but I have always had difficulty in understanding the mechanism and in distinguishing it from intermittent claudication.
Consultant	I appreciate your difficulty since both conditions are based on ischaemia. In spinal stenosis it is the spinal arteries that are involved and produce ischaemia affecting the cauda equina of the spinal cord. The cause of the arterial insufficiency is marked narrowing of the spinal canal in the lower part of the vertebral column by either extensive osteoarthritic changes or sometimes by congenital narrowing. The ischaemia of the cauda equina is precipitated by walking and results in the development of neurological symptoms like numbness, tingling or muscle weakness. Have you any idea how you would distinguish it from intermittent claudication?
Student	I suppose that you would be more likely to find evidence of extensive arteriosclerosis in the patient with claudication.
Consultant	Yes that is a good point. Any others?
Student	As we mentioned earlier, spinal stenosis produces neurological symptoms while claudication causes mainly pain in the legs.
Consultant	What about the site of the pain in the two conditions?
Student	Well, I know that claudication pain usually involves the calves, but I'm not sure with spinal stenosis.
Consultant	It usually affects the thighs and often the patient's back as well, but we must also remember that claudication can produce pain in the thighs in some circumstances; do you know which?
Student	If the arterial obstruction is high up in the aorta or in the iliac arteries.

Consultant	Good. I'll just mention the other differentiating points since I doubt that you will be familiar with them. The pain in spinal stenosis is provoked more often walking downhill unlike claudication which is worse uphill, and relief of symptoms in spinal stenosis can occur by flexing the spine whereas claudication is eased only by stopping the walking. One final and obvious point in spinal stenosis is that <u>bladder and bowel symptoms may occur which never happens with claudication</u>. I hope you now feel adequately enlightened on spinal stenosis! We must return to Mr M.'s problems. Can you think of any other possible diagnoses?
Student	I did think of myasthenia gravis as an alternative diagnosis in view of the development of the leg symptoms after exertion.
Consultant	An interesting suggestion! Does he have any other symptoms to indicate myasthenia gravis?
Student	I didn't actually ask him specifically about this.
Consultant	If a patient's history suggests any possible diagnoses to you — which it always should do — you should follow it up by asking specific questions in relation to these diagnoses. Ask Mr M. now about other symptoms of myasthenia gravis.
Student	Mr M., do you have any difficulty in chewing or swallowing?
Patient	I can't say that I have ever noticed any.
Student	Do you have any weakness in your arms after you have been using them for any length of time?
Patient	I haven't had any trouble with my arms either.
Student	I don't think that he has myasthenia.
Consultant	You've asked the right questions but you could also have asked him about drooping of the eyelids, double vision and weakening of his voice after he has been speaking for a time. I would agree with you, however, that myasthenia gravis is not the diagnosis. What other neurological conditions should we think of to explain Mr M.'s walking difficulties?
Student	We've already suggested that he has spastic legs so we must consider the likely causes of spasticity.
Consultant	Yes, I agree with that proposition. <u>Tell me first what part of his nervous system is involved to lead to spasticity?</u>
Student	It is due to a lesion of the pyramidal tracts.
Consultant	Good. What type of lesion do you have in mind?
Student	One condition which I think we should consider is demyelination.
Consultant	You mean multiple sclerosis. Is there anything else in the history which would support that diagnosis?
Student	I thought that the blurring of vision might be due to retro-bulbar neuritis.
Consultant	Yes, that is certainly a possibility. Did he have any pain behind the eye

when his vision was blurred because this would be strong supporting evidence of retro-bulbar neuritis?

Student   I didn't ask him.

Consultant   Would you like to ask him now?

Student   Mr M., did you notice any pain or aching behind your eye when you had these episodes of blurred vision?

Patient   Now that you mention it, I have had aching in the eye at the same time as I had difficulty in reading because of the blurring, but I put this down to eye-strain.

Consultant   This is suggestive of retro-bulbar neuritis. What causes do you know apart from MS?

Student   The only other cause I can remember is alcoholism.

Consultant   Yes, that can be a cause, and it may also occur in diabetes — not very common in my experience — vitamin B_1 and B_{12} deficiency, tobacco poisoning and we mustn't forget good old-fashioned neurosyphilis — very rare nowadays but prevalent when I was a student.

Let's get back to the spastic legs. Are there any other causes that we should consider for this?

Student   It can certainly occur with cerebrovascular disease.

Consultant   Can you be a bit more specific?

Student   What I had in mind was some form of stroke.

Consultant   What part of the brain is affected in a stroke to cause spasticity?

Student   It's usually due to involvement of the internal capsule.

Consultant   That is correct, but the involvement is almost invariably unilateral. As I understand it, Mr M. has trouble with both legs. Are there any sites in the brain where a vascular lesion can produce bilateral pyramidal involvement of the legs?

Student   Yes, I think this would happen if he had a lesion in the brain-stem.

Consultant   That would do it but wouldn't you find other symptoms as well?

Student   You would expect involvement of other structures in the brain stem.

Consultant   If I were to ask you to detail the specific 'structures' would you be able to do so?

Student   I doubt it.

Consultant   OK, I won't put you to the test now but what I want you to do is to draw a diagram of a cross-section of the brain-stem and let us all see it at the next ward round (Figure 10.1).

Can you think of any other causes of pyramidal involvement in a young man of 33?

Student   What about subacute combined degeneration of the spinal cord?

Consultant   What is the usual cause of this condition?

Student	Pernicious anaemia.
Consultant	And is it likely that a patient of this age would develop pernicious anaemia?
Student	Very unlikely, I think.
Consultant	I would agree with you, except perhaps in two instances. One is if the patient for any reason has had a resection of a particular part of the bowel. Which part?
Student	The terminal ileum, because that is the area where vitamin B_{12} is absorbed.
Consultant	Well done! Strictly speaking, that would not really be pernicious anaemia, would it?
Student	No, because pernicious anaemia is due to a failure of production of the intrinsic factor by the stomach while resection of the ileum just leads to a failure to absorb B_{12}.
Consultant	Now, what is the other circumstance in which a young man may develop a B_{12}-deficiency anaemia?
Student	I don't know.
Consultant	Chronic alcoholism, but Mr M.'s modest intake of alcohol excludes this possibility. Can you think of any other causes of pyramidal involvement?
Student	He could have pressure on the spinal cord by a neoplasm.
Consultant	Yes, that is another possibility. If that was the problem you'd expect other symptoms, wouldn't you?
Student	I would expect him to have some sensory symptoms as well as motor symptoms involving the legs.
Consultant	A spinal cord lesion of this type would be very likely to involve other long tracts, so sensory symptoms would be almost inevitable. Additionally, he ought to have bladder symptoms which is common with spinal cord pressure. Since Mr M. has neither sensory nor urinary symptoms, the diagnosis is unlikely, but it is obviously something you should focus on when you present your examination findings. Any other causes?
Student	Could he have a space-occupying lesion in the brain?
Consultant	This could of course affect the pyramidal tracts, but do you think this is a likely possibility and how would you decide?
Student	He doesn't complain of any headache which makes a space-occupying lesion unlikely.
Consultant	Yes, I think that is an important point. Headache is often an early manifestation of raised intracranial pressure and you would expect it in a patient with a space-occupying lesion. Is there anything else for or against this diagnosis?
Student	Presumably he would have other neurological symptoms, especially fits.

Consultant	I would agree with this. Isolated pyramidal tract involvement as a result of a space-occupying lesion in the brain is, in my experience, extremely rare. Have you heard of Friedreich's* ataxia?
Student	I've heard of it but I can't remember much about it apart from the fact that it is a hereditary disorder and it is associated with some cardiac abnormality.
Consultant	That's very good. It is a hereditary degenerative disease affecting the spino-cerebellar and pyramidal tracts: the main clinical manifestations are unsteadiness and spastic weakness of the legs, and up to 90% have ECG abnormalities, mainly heart block. This is another diagnosis, therefore, we ought to keep in mind when we examine him. I'll mention one final diagnosis to consider in a patient with spastic legs — motor neurone disease. What do you think of this suggestion?
Student	I thought that it always produced muscle atrophy and a flaccid paralysis, not a spastic one.
Consultant	You are quite right. Motor neurone degeneration in the anterior horns of the spinal cord produces flaccid paralysis, as in progressive muscular atrophy affecting the hands or bulbar palsy involving the cranial nerves. But another component of the disease is degeneration of the pyramidal cells in the brain leading to spasticity as in amyotrophic lateral sclerosis. The combination of muscle wasting, flaccid paralysis and Babinski[†] responses should always suggest the possibility of motor neurone disease. I think the time has now come to summarize our conclusions from the history:

> HISTORY
>
> - we think Mr M. has pyramidal tract involvement leading to spasticity of the legs
> - his episodes of blurred vision might be due to retro-bulbar neuritis
> - the combination of pyramidal involvement and retro-bulbar neuritis makes it likely that he has multiple sclerosis
> - the other possible diagnoses we need to keep in mind include a spinal cord tumour and hereditary spino-cerebellar ataxia

Consultant	Would you like to present your examination findings now, and could I suggest that you begin with the nervous system since we think that is where the problem lies.

* N. Friedreich (1825–1882), a German neurologist, was Professor of Pathology in Heidelberg.
† J.F.F. Babinski (1857–1932), of Polish extraction, who graduated in Paris and worked with the famous French neurologist, Charcot. Babinski was the first to introduce the technique of kneeling the patient to elicit the knee jerk.

Student	I'll start with his legs.
Consultant	Why not start with the cranial nerves?
Student	Because his symptoms are primarily concerned with his legs.
Consultant	All right, that's a reasonable answer. I'm glad to see that you are grasping the essential requirement in a clinical examination of concentrating on 'where the action is'. Please carry on.
Student	There was normal tone in the legs but there is definite weakness of the right leg affecting mainly flexion of the thigh and dorsiflexion of the foot.
Consultant	I'm glad that you tested power thoroughly by assessing flexion and extension at all the joints — hips, knees and feet. Sometimes students miss out on the full range of movements. I agree with your findings on the weakness of the right lower limb, but not with your comment on normal tone.

The consultant abruptly lifts both of the patient's legs in turn from under the thigh — it is obvious that the right leg is stiffer than the left indicating spasticity.

Consultant	Would you like to carry on with your examination of the legs?
Student	Pin-prick and cotton wool sensation . . .
Consultant	Why have you gone from the motor system to the sensory system? Haven't you left something out?
Student	I'll come back to the reflexes in a moment.
Consultant	I suggest you come back to them now. You must try to be systematic. When examining the motor system start with a comment on muscle wasting and fasciculation — both of which incidentally you omitted — then you go on to muscle tone, power and reflexes, including plantar response. Don't switch backwards and forwards from the motor system to the sensory system. Before you continue with your examination let me ask you whether wasting and fasciculation could be relevant in Mr M.?
Student	It would indicate the possibility of motor neurone disease, which was in our differential diagnosis, so it is relevant. He doesn't show either.
Consultant	Carry on with your examination.
Student	His reflexes were brisk in both legs.
Consultant	Do you mean normally brisk or abnormally brisk? The term 'brisk' is used often to avoid making a clinical decision as to whether reflexes are abnormally increased or not. Reliable judgement on this will come with experience but the first step is at least to try to make up your mind.
Student	I think that the reflexes are increased abnormally and I also think that the right side is brisker than the left.

Consultant	I agree. There is another simple test you can do which might help in confirming that the reflexes are abnormally brisk.
Student	Do you mean the plantar responses?
Consultant	That is obviously very important and we will come to it in a moment but not the test I had in mind.
Student	I'm not sure then what you mean.
Consultant	I'm referring to ankle clonus. Did you test for this?
Student	No, I'm sorry I forgot. I'll check it now.

The student demonstrates sustained clonus on abruptly flexing the patient's right ankle. It is not present on the left.

Consultant	Now you can tell us about the plantar responses.
Student	The right Babinski is positive but I wasn't sure on the left.
Consultant	Let me remind you of one important thing about the Babinski response and clear up a common misconception among students. The Babinski response is not synonymous with the plantar response; the Babinski response means an *extensor* plantar response so it is either present or absent. Have I made it clear?
Student	Yes, thank you. Mr M. has a Babinski response on the right but the left side is equivocal.

The consultant tests the plantar responses and both big toes go up on the first stroke of the soles.

Consultant	I don't think that I will try it again — I might get a normal plantar response the next time! We now seem to have good evidence of pyramidal involvement in the right leg and probably the left leg also. Can you think of any other tests for pyramidal damage?
Student	I don't do any other tests.
Consultant	When I was a student we were taught always to check the superficial abdominal reflexes which disappear if the pyramidal tracts are damaged. The other test we used to do was the cremasteric reflex which you have probably never heard of, have you?
Student	I'm afraid I don't know the cremasteric reflex but I am aware of the superficial abdominal reflex.
Consultant	These reflexes may be of help when you are doubtful about the presence of pyramidal changes. The cremasteric reflex involves stroking the inside of the thigh which normally causes retraction of the testis on that side — a reflex lost if pyramidal damage is present. One word of advice though with this reflex — do make sure that you have a patient of the right sex otherwise you may find yourself up before the General

Medical Council! Would you like to try it — sister is holding out an orange stick for you.

The student tries the cremasteric reflex on both sides and seems inordinately pleased when he finds an absent response on the right side.

Consultant   Well done. This confirms the pyramidal involvement on the right side. Would you like to try the abdominal reflexes now? One little appeal though; do try not to leave the patient's abdomen a mass of linear wheals by repeated attempts at eliciting the reflex — one try should be enough.

All the superficial reflexes are absent.

Consultant   The absent reflexes on the two sides confirms our view that Mr M. has bilateral pyramidal involvement. This seems to be a more sensitive indicator of pyramidal involvement in Mr M. than the cremasteric reflex.
    Would you like to tell us about the sensory findings now?

Student   I found that pin-prick was unaffected but there is definite impairment of joint position sense in the right foot.

Consultant   What does this mean?

Student   He probably has posterior column involvement.

Consultant   Did you do any other tests of posterior column function?

Student   Yes, his vibration sense was reduced at the ankle on the right but cotton wool sensation seemed normal.

Consultant   Why is this if we say that light touch (cotton wool) is carried in the posterior columns?

Student   I think that some light touch fibres are also carried in other tracts in the spinal cord.

Consultant   Good. Dare I ask you which?

Student   I'm not sure.

Consultant   The lateral spino-thalamic tract, which gives me another bright idea. Would you like to draw us a cross-section of the spinal cord as well as the brain-stem?

Student   Not really but I'll have a go.

Consultant   I think it will be a salutary and informative experience for you and indeed for all of us when you show us the diagrams (Figure 10.2).
    Do you think that this evidence of posterior column involvement, when considered in association with the pyramidal tract damage, helps us in deciding the diagnosis?

Student   It could indicate subacute combined degeneration of the spinal cord.

Consultant   I think that we have already agreed that this is an unlikely diagnosis in view of his age.

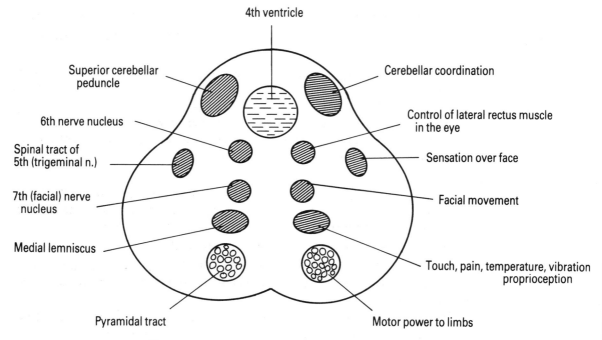

Figure 10.1 Transverse section through the pons.

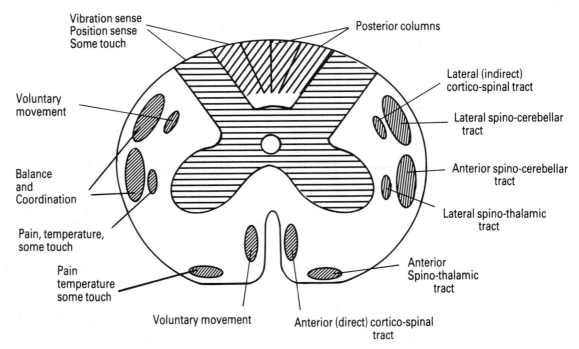

Figure 10.2 Transverse section of the spinal cord.

Student	Then I think that the next diagnosis to consider is multiple sclerosis.
Consultant	I would agree that comes high on the list. What about motor neurone disease?
Student	No, it is not motor neurone disease because you don't get posterior column changes and also Mr M. does not show any muscle wasting or fasciculation.
Consultant	Could the signs indicate Friedreich's ataxia? We've already said that you get involvement of the pyramidal tracts and posterior columns in Friedreich's ataxia.
Student	I suppose this still remains a possibility.
Consultant	You have not yet told us about Mr M.'s cerebellar function in the legs. This would obviously be very relevant in Friedreich's ataxia because this is the other main tract affected, the spino-cerebellar tract.
Student	I thought that his heel–knee test was normal.
Consultant	This would be against the diagnosis. Since you are presenting your findings in reverse order, perhaps you had better tell us now about the upper limbs.
Student	I found no abnormality in either the motor or sensory systems but he wasn't very good at the finger–nose test on the left side.
Consultant	What does this suggest?
Student	That his cerebellar function is impaired on this side.
Consultant	There is another test of cerebellar function that all students love to roll their tongues around.
Student	You mean adiadochokinesis?
Consultant	That's the one. Have you tried it?
Student	I did in fact and thought that it was abnormal.

The student demonstrates the finger–nose test which was obviously impaired on the left, and follows it up by showing convincing difficulty by the patient in rapid supination/pronation movements at the left wrist compared with the right.

Consultant	Well, you have convinced us all by that demonstration. Does he have any symptoms relating to this incoordination in the left arm?
Student	I don't think so.
Consultant	Mr M. have you noticed any problems in using your left arm or left hand?
Patient	Funny you should ask that. I have noticed recently that my left arm has been a bit clumsy — I seem to drop things with this arm which I never did before.
Consultant	That is very likely due to his cerebellar impairment. I think we had better

proceed now to the cranial nerves. What would you particularly look for if you were considering a demyelinating disorder?

Student   You would examine the optic discs for evidence of optic atrophy.

Consultant   What would this signify?

Student   That he has had retro-bulbar neuritis in the past.

Consultant   And does he show optic atrophy?

Student   I'm not sure. I thought that he might show some pallor on the temporal side of both discs, but I always have difficulty in deciding whether it is pathological.

Consultant   A difficulty shared by many I can assure you. It will get easier with experience. I would agree that the lateral side of the discs is a little pale but I would regard it as within normal limits. If he did have optic atrophy I think the pallor would be much more marked. Were there any other abnormal findings in the cranial nerves?

Student   No, I thought that all the other nerves were intact.

Consultant   That completes your examination of the nervous system. What are your final conclusions from this examination?

Student   I think that the findings point to multiple sclerosis.

Consultant   Why do you say that?

Student   He has evidence of involvement of the pyramidal tracts, posterior columns and the cerebellar tracts.

Consultant   What you are quite rightly saying is that you have found disseminated lesions in the spinal cord which is of course the diagnostic feature of multiple sclerosis, or to give it perhaps the more apt old-fashioned name, disseminated sclerosis — lesions disseminated both in space and time. The past history of blurred vision suggesting retrobulbar neuritis gives you the dissemination in time.

                 Before we proceed to the investigation of the nervous system I should ask you whether you found any abnormality on examination of any of the other systems?

Student   No, I think the rest of the examination was normal.

Consultant   The only other finding we might perhaps have expected is some evidence of chronic bronchitis in view of the smoking. Fortunately Mr M.'s lungs appear to be all right now but I doubt if they will stay that way if he goes on smoking.

Patient   I'm going to have another go at giving up. I haven't had any since I came into hospital.

Consultant   Was it Mark Twain* who said giving up smoking is easy — he has done it many times!

* Mark Twain, a pseudonym for Samuel Clemens (1835–1910), was a famous American humorist and author.

Perhaps we could now summarize our conclusions from the examination findings:

> ### EXAMINATION
> - there is evidence of bilateral pyramidal involvement though most of the signs affect the right leg
> - there is posterior column involvement in the right leg
> - there is evience of mild cerebellar involvement in the left arm
> - the optic discs do not show atrophy
> - the combination of pyramidal, posterior column and cerebellar signs suggest that the most likely diagnosis is disseminated sclerosis

Now, let me ask you about investigating Mr M. What tests do you think might be useful?

Student	The first test we should do is a lumbar puncture.
Consultant	That's a good suggestion. What do you hope to find?
Student	It might give us some evidence of MS.
Consultant	Like what?
Student	The protein would be increased, especially the gamma-globulin.
Consultant	That's right. When I was a student we always used to do another special test on the CSF — it was called the Lange test; it involved precipitation of CSF protein by colloidal gold solution. The dilutions at which precipitation occurs give diagnostic pointers to conditions like MS (paretic curve), tabes dorsalis (luetic curve) and meningitis (meningitic curve). Nowadays we have more sophisticated techniques applied to the CSF like electrophoresis which shows IgG in at least 90% of patients with MS. Do you know any other useful tests for diagnosing multiple sclerosis?
Student	I can't think of any other tests.
Consultant	Have you heard of the visual-evoked reflex?
Student	Yes, I have. It's something to do with the electroencephalogram but I don't know any other details.
Consultant	It is based on showing slower conduction in the optic nerves due to demyelination. It involves shining a light in the patient's eyes and recording the time taken for the arrival of the impulse in the occipital cortex. It's a very useful test in picking up MS, even when the patient has not had any obvious clinical episodes of retro-bulbar neuritis. I should perhaps add that it is not pathognomic for MS; the response time can also be prolonged in glaucoma, optic nerve compression by tumour and other forms of optic neuritis. There is one other very new type of investigation which offers great potential in diagnosing MS.

Student	I think I know the answer to that one — CT brain scan.
Consultant	That's a very good try. It's not CT scanning which I have in mind because it's unlikely to be sensitive enough to show up the MS lesions in the brain. The other better investigation, allied to CT scanning, is nuclear magnetic resonance which can show changes in the chemical composition of the nerve fibres and so pick up demyelination. NMR is not readily available yet because it involves very expensive equipment. Now, what about the other diagnoses we considered earlier? You remember we discussed a space-occupying lesion of the spinal cord, subacute combined degeneration of the spinal cord and Friedreich's ataxia — would any tests help in these conditions?
Student	A serum B_{12} level would tell us about subacute combined degeneration.
Consultant	I'm glad you asked for the B_{12} level rather than the blood count because the neurological manifestations of B_{12} deficiency can occur in the absence of anaemia. What about a spinal cord lesion?
Student	I think that a CT scan of the spinal cord would help.
Consultant	I would agree that this is probably the best test, though the more conventional and also very useful test is . . . ·
Student	Myelography.
Consultant	That's right. What about Friedreich's ataxia?
Student	The ECG might show conduction disturbances as we mentioned earlier.
Consultant	That's so, but we must remember that these changes are very non-specific. I think we both agree that the most likely diagnosis is multiple sclerosis so that these other investigations are probably unnecessary anyway. I might stress perhaps at this point that even if the CSF analysis and the visual-evoked reflex are normal I would still not exclude multiple sclerosis and I would think it worthwhile to set up a therapeutic trial of either a 3-week course of intramuscular ACTH or a week's course of intravenous methyl prednisolone — a favourable response would support a diagnosis of MS.

OUTCOME

Mr M.'s CSF result was:

		Normal range
Cells	8 lymphocytes/mm^3	up to 4/mm^3
Total protein	120 mg/100 ml	up to 40 mg/100 ml
Gamma-globulin	22 mg/100 ml	up to 5 mg/100 ml

This result is very suggestive of multiple sclerosis, and the diagnosis was confirmed by finding impaired conduction in both optic nerves in the visual-evoked reflex.

The patient was given a week's course of intravenous methyl prednisolone and intensive physiotherapy. He improved considerably in the power in the right leg though the signs of pyramidal damage remained. Physiotherapy was arranged after discharge as long as he continued to make further progress.

NB Prognosis of multiple sclerosis

Seventy per cent of patients will improve after the initial event. About 50% will be able to continue work and domestic commitments 10 years after onset.

Twenty-five per cent of patients will remain active for 20 years.

Favourable prognostic features

Onset < 40 years
Onset with retro-bulbar neuritis
Long interval between attacks
Infrequent attacks

Unfavourable prognostic features

Onset > 40 years
Onset with brain-stem involvement
Less than 1 year between first and second attacks
Frequent relapses

LEARNING POINTS

Causes of pyramidal tract disease

- cerebrovascular disease
- multiple sclerosis
- spinal cord compression e.g. tumour
- subacute combined degeneration
- motor neurone disease
- vascular lesions of the spinal cord

Signs of pyramidal disease

- muscle weakness
- increased reflexes
- ankle clonus
- Babinski response
- absent superficial abdominal reflex
- absent cremasteric reflex
- spastic gait — toe catching

Causes of combined posterior column and pyramidal tract involvement

- multiple sclerosis
- subacute combined degeneration
- Friedreich's ataxia
- syphilitic tabo-paresis

Features of Friedreich's ataxia

- posterior column involvement
    loss of reflexes
    loss of vibration and joint-position sense
- pyramidal involvement
    increased reflexes
    Babinski response
- spino-cerebellar tracts
    severe ataxia
- other organs
    spina bifida
    scoliosis
    pes cavus
    heart block
    cardiomyopathy

Types of motor neurone disease

- bulbar palsy
- progressive muscular atrophy
- amyotrophic lateral sclerosis

Features of brain-stem lesion

- bilateral pyramidal involvement
- bilateral sensory changes in the limbs
- cranial nerve involvement
- involvement of the cerebellar tracts

Causes of retro-bulbar neuritis

- multiple sclerosis
- diabetes mellitus
- vitamin deficiency
    B_1
    B_{12}
- syphilis
- toxins
    lead
    alcohol
    quinine
    tobacco

Diagnostic tests in multiple sclerosis

- CSF
    gamma-globulin increased
    mild lymphocytosis (10–15)
    paretic Lange curve
- visual-evoked reflex
    slow conduction in optic nerve
- nuclear magnetic resonance
    chemical changes of demyelination
- therapeutic trial of steroid treatment

Differentiation between claudication and spinal stenosis

Claudication	*Spinal stenosis*
Foot pulses reduced or absent	Foot pulses present
Pain usually in calf but may involve thighs/buttocks	Pain in back and thighs — rarely in calves
Walking produces pain	Walking produces pain, weakness and paraesthesiae
Worse going uphill	Worse going downhill
Relieved on resting	Relief with rest but also with stretching back
No bladder/bowel symptoms	Bladder/bowel symptoms common

11

Back pain

Student	Mrs B.N. is a 61-year-old housewife who has been admitted to hospital because she has been losing weight and feeling very tired. She has lost about one stone over the last 3 or 4 months and she thinks this is because she has been off her food and not eating — she says her appetite has been very poor lately. Over the same period she has noticed that she gets tired very easily. She always had plenty of energy before and had been able to cope with her housework as well as a part-time cleaning job in an office, but now she feels everything is such an effort and she has had to give up her cleaning job and finds it takes all her time just to keep up with her housework.
	Her other complaint relates to her back. She has had a lot of trouble with her back over the years and it seems to be getting much worse recently. The pain in her back is in the lower part of her spine and sometimes goes down her left leg. She has seen an orthopaedic specialist and he told her that she had 'arthritis of the spine'. During the last few months her back has been giving her a lot of pain but the pain seems to be higher up in the spine than her usual pain, and isn't settling down as quickly as it used to do.
	There were no other serious illnesses in the past, though she did mention a 'minor' operation on her womb about 3 years ago which she was apparently advised to have after she had a cervical smear; she's not too sure what was done but she thinks it had something to do with the neck of the womb.
	She is a long-standing smoker, about 20 to 25 cigarettes a day since she was 20 years old and she has tried to give up on a number of occasions without much success. She has a chronic smoker's cough but has very little phlegm at present.
	I couldn't get anything significant in the family history.
Consultant	Would you start by telling us what you thought of the history?
Student	Her main complaints were the loss of weight and the severe tiredness.
Consultant	You have already told us that, but what I want from you is possible causes for her symptoms.
Student	Mrs N. thinks that her loss of weight is because her appetite has been poor and she has not been eating much.

Consultant	That's no answer is it? The important question is why her appetite has become so poor.
Student	There are a lot of causes of a poor appetite.
Consultant	Would you like to tell us some of these causes?
Student	At this age I suppose one of the first conditions to think of would be a neoplasm.
Consultant	That's a good suggestion and neoplasm is of prime importance in the differential diagnosis. If Mrs N. is suffering from a neoplastic condition, where would you think the neoplasm is likely to be?
Student	The stomach would be a likely site.
Consultant	Yes, this is one of the more common sites leading to anorexia, but it is important to remember that a neoplasm anywhere can and often is associated with anorexia and loss of weight, so we must keep an open mind. Any other causes of anorexia?
Student	You can get it with a gastric ulcer.
Consultant	The lack of eating in gastric ulcer is not a true anorexia — it is because the patient is afraid to eat as food often leads to pain. Can you suggest any other conditions associated with anorexia.
Student	Do you get it in uraemia?
Consultant	Yes, chronic renal failure is certainly a cause. Anything else?
Student	I can't think of any more just at the moment.
Consultant	It might be helpful to divide the causes of loss of appetite into gastro-intestinal causes, like gastric neoplasm which you have already mentioned, hepatitis, pancreatitis and inflammatory bowel disease, endocrine disorders like Addison's* disease, myxoedema and hyperparathyroidism, neoplasia and chronic renal failure which we also mentioned earlier, and finally, don't forget drugs, the main one causing anorexia being . . .
Student	I don't know.

Consultant	Digitalis, especially in elderly patients.
	    Now, if I may, I would like to shift the emphasis of the questioning back to the causes of loss of weight rather than the causes of anorexia, since I think this is the real worry that Mrs N. has, though obviously some of the conditions we have already mentioned are common to both.
	    Can you think, therefore, of any other causes of loss of weight that we haven't covered?

* Thomas Addison (1793–1860) was a physician at Guy's Hospital and a contemporary of Thomas Hodgkin and Richard Bright. He published his famous monograph 'On the Constitutional and Local Effects of Disease of the Supra-renal Capsule' in 1855. He also described pernicious anaemia.

Student	What about thyrotoxicosis?
Consultant	That's a good one, especially in an elderly patient where other helpful manifestations of thyrotoxicosis may not be very obvious — a condition often called 'masked' thyrotoxicosis. Did you follow up this possibility by direct questioning?
Student	No, I didn't think of this diagnosis at the time I was taking Mrs. N.'s history.
Consultant	It is important to train yourself to react to symptoms in every patient by thinking of likely causes at the time you are taking the history, and then follow up by asking appropriate questions in relation to those diagnoses to get an idea whether the diagnosis is a feasible one. Would you like to ask Mrs N. any questions to help you decide whether she might have thyrotoxicosis?
Student	Mrs N., can you tell us whether you prefer could weather to hot weather.
Consultant	Before Mrs N. answers that question, you don't really think we are going to let you get away with the way you have put it? You must phrase it in a more neutral manner and give her a proper choice of telling you the weather she prefers.
Student	I'm sorry. Mrs N., can you tell us whether you have any special preference for either hot weather or cold weather?
Patient	It doesn't make much difference to me either way, though I do like it hot when I go away on holiday.
Consultant	Do you have any other questions for her?
Student	Mrs N., could I ask you also whether you have any palpitations or if you sweat excessively?
Patient	No, I don't suffer with palpitations except if I rush about — and I can't do much of that nowadays — and I don't think I sweat more than normal.
Student	What about your nerves — do you think these are getting bad?
Patient	Well, I have been very depressed lately because I feel so useless.
Consultant	I have not found that asking about a patient's nerves has been of much help in diagnosing thyrotoxicosis. There is one other symptom which is against this diagnosis also — do you know what symptom?
Student	A poor appetite would be very unusual in a thyrotoxic patient.
Consultant	That's right. I think we both agree that thyrotoxicosis is a very unlikely diagnosis. Can you tell us any other endocrine causes of loss of weight?
Student	Loss of weight occurs in diabetes.
Consultant	Yes, that is a major symptom in the diagnosis of diabetes; what are the other two cardinal symptoms?

Student	Polyuria and polydipsia.
Consultant	Good — did you ask Mrs N. about these symptoms?
Student	No, I'm afraid I didn't.
Consultant	You must try to follow up all the possible diagnoses you think of when you are taking the history, as I mentioned earlier — this can't be emphasized too often! Would you like to ask her now?
Student	Mrs N., can you tell us whether you have noticed any change in the amount of water you are passing, or whether you have been feeling excessively thirsty?
Patient	I have noticed that I have to get up at night recently to go to the toilet, but I can't say that I am more thirsty than usual.
Consultant	The recent nocturia might be relevant, and we will come back to this later. Can you think of any other causes of loss of weight that we ought to consider — let me give you a clue about one cause which is often forgotten; it occurs in patients with certain types of heart disease.
Student	Do you mean heart failure?
Consultant	No, that is not what I had in mind, though I think it only fair to admit that chronic heart failure can be associated with quite considerable weight loss — a condition known as cardiac cachexia. The cardiac condition I was thinking of is an infective one — that will give it away.
Student	You mean subacute bacterial endocarditis?
Consultant	That's right. Infective endocarditis — which is the better term — may cause anorexia and loss of weight and often very little else in the way of symptoms. What type of heart disease would you expect to be associated with infective endocarditis?
Student	Rheumatic heart disease.
Consultant	Yes, that is the most frequent but you mustn't forget congenital heart disease also. Has Mrs N. anything in her history to suggest the possibility of rheumatic heart disease?
Student	She didn't mention any heart problems.
Consultant	Did you ask her about rheumatic fever or St Vitus' dance?
Student	No, I didn't, but there is no evidence of rheumatic heart disease on examination.
Consultant	We are still concentrating on the history, so your examination findings are not relevant at this point. Asking about rheumatic fever, St Vitus' dance and even 'growing pains' used to be a standard question when I was a student because

	rheumatic heart disease was such a common problem; nowadays I suppose the only contact that some students will have with rheumatic heart disease is in their examination finals!
	Incidentally, who was St Vitus?
Student	I have no idea.
Consultant	Obviously, your teachers are not as holy as in my day! St Vitus was the patron saint of dancing, and if you have ever seen a child with rheumatic chorea you will realize why the condition was called St Vitus' dance.
	Are there any other types of infection which we should think of which could cause a profound loss of weight?
Student	I can't think of any more common infections.
Consultant	We mustn't forget tuberculosis. What other symptoms might you expect in this condition?
Student	If it affected the lungs I would expect a cough and sputum, quite possibly with haemoptysis.
Consultant	Good, but don't forget that tuberculosis can affect other systems apart from the lungs, like the lymph glands or the bowel. There is one distinctive symptom which is common to all forms of tuberculosis.
Student	I'm not sure what it is.
Consultant	You probably don't see much tuberculosis now, unlike my student days when it was quite rife. I'm referring to bouts of profuse sweating, especially at night.
	Mrs N. has nothing like this, so I think we can move on.
	At this juncture I think we should now turn to Mrs N.'s other important problem — her back pain. What are your thoughts on this?
Student	It sounds like osteo-arthritis of the spine, perhaps with some disc trouble as well.
Consultant	I would agree that the most likely diagnosis of her chronic back problem is osteoarthritis and the radiation down her leg suggests root involvement. Don't you think that her recent pain might be different?
Student	Well, she has noticed some differences — it is higher up in the back and it seems to be more persistent.
Consultant	Was the onset sudden or gradual?
Student	I didn't ask her that. Mrs N., how did your recent back pain start — was it suddenly?
Patient	Well, now you mention it, it did seem to come on all at once — I was in the garden doing some weeding when it came on. I thought it was my old back trouble again because I have had that once or twice when I've been bending down in the garden, but this pain seemed in a different place.
Consultant	(To student) Did you ask her any other details about her recent pain —

	where exactly it is and whether there are any aggravating or relieving factors? This may give you some useful clues as to its cause.
Student	No, I'm sorry, I didn't go into much detail with Mrs N. Mrs N., when do you get the back pain — what brings it on?
Patient	The pain seems to be there all the time.
Consultant	(To patient) Do you get the pain in bed, Mrs N.?
Patient	It's even worse in bed. I sometimes have to get out of bed to get some relief, though it never seems to leave me for long.
Consultant	Was that the same with your other back pain?
Patient	No, it's quite different. Previously I used to get pain when I was moving about, especially when I was bending or lifting something, and I was able to get relief by resting in bed. With this pain I don't seem to get any relief.
Consultant	(To student) I think you will agree that Mrs N.'s present back pain is quite different to her previous pain. What do you think this could be due to?
Student	Could it be due to osteo-arthritis higher up in the dorsal spine?
Consultant	In my experience, osteo-arthritis of the dorsal spine rarely causes much in the way of symptoms and never severe and persistent pain like Mrs N. has.
Student	Then I think that the other possibility is neoplasia.
Consultant	What type of neoplasia.
Student	She could have a mitotic deposit.
Consultant	Yes, I should think that would come high on the list. Is there anything in the history which might support that suggestion?
Student	Well, one possibility would be that it is related to the problem she had with her uterus.
Consultant	That's a reasonable suggestion. Anything else significant in the history?
Student	I don't think so.
Consultant	What about the smoking?
Student	I'm sorry, I forgot about that. It could certainly be relevant if she had a primary lesion in the bronchus.
Consultant	That is obviously another possibility that we will have to keep very much in mind.
	Is there any other form of neoplasia which might affect the spine?
Student	Myelomatosis.
Consultant	Yes, that is also a very important diagnosis to consider. In relation to this possibility, I wonder if you would like to make any comments about her nocturia.

Student	I'm not too sure what you are getting at.
Consultant	If the nocturia is an early manifestation of renal failure, what I am asking is whether there could be any relationship between renal failure and myelomatosis?
Student	Myeloma can affect the kidneys.
Consultant	Not only 'can' but often does, and this involvement is the most likely reason if the prognosis turns out to be adverse. The nocturia, then, would lend some support to the possibility of myelomatosis in Mrs N. Now, can I have your thoughts on Mrs N.'s other main symptom, the extreme tiredness — why is she so tired?
Student	I think the reason she is so tired is because she is anaemic.
Consultant	Why do you say that?
Student	Because she looks very pale.
Consultant	Fair enough! Her pallor will obviously register with you when you are taking the history, and so it should. Why is Mrs N. anaemic?
Student	It could be due to neoplasia.
consultant	It could indeed in her case because there are some other pointers to this diagnosis. If she didn't have the other clues, what diagnoses would you think of to account for her anaemia?
Student	Blood loss would be the most likely cause.
Consultant	Bleeding from where?
Student	The gastro-intestinal tract would be the commonest site.
Consultant	That's right. When you saw Mrs N. was obviously anaemic, did you ask her about any likely causes in the gastro-intestinal tract which might be responsible for bleeding?
Student	I asked about indigestion — she doesn't have any.
Consultant	Peptic ulcer is one of the commonest causes of GI bleeding. What about the other end of the GI tract — does she have any history of piles?
Student	I didn't ask her.
Consultant	It's one of the most important questions to ask if you suspect bleeding from the GI tract.
Patient	I don't suffer with piles as far as I know.
Consultant	Is there any other question you should ask if you think there is GI bleeding?
Student	Whether the patient has taken any drugs like the non-steroidal anti-inflammatory agents.
Consultant	And has she?

Student	She may have — she told me she had taken a lot of tablets to try to relieve her back pain.
Consultant	Then that is another possible cause for us to keep in mind to account for the anaemia. Incidentally, don't forget that steroids also cause gastro-intestinal bleeding as well as the non-steroidal drugs — and don't forget aspirin also as a cause of bleeding, probably one of the commonest causes of all. Any other GI causes of bleeding?
Student	It could be due to a mitotic lesion of the GI tract.
Consultant	Where would be the likely site?
Student	In the caecum.
Consultant	Yes, this frequently presents with anaemia; similarly with lesions elsewhere in the ascending colon. Another common site for neoplastic bleeding would be in the stomach. Can you think of any more gastro-intestinal lesions causing bleeding?
Student	I can't think of any others at the moment.
Consultant	If I told you it was related to drinking?
Student	Do you mean alcoholic gastritis.
Consultant	No, that is not what I had in mind and I don't think that is likely to be a major cause of blood loss. I'm thinking of a condition occurring in the oesophagus as a result of chronic heavy drinking.
Student	Oh, you mean oesophageal varices.
Consultant	That's right — it's surprising how often that is forgotten when I ask students about the causes of gastro-intestinal bleeding. Now, two other important causes of anaemia, especially in the elderly — what are these?
Student	Pernicious anaemia.
Consultant	Good. What is the other one?
Student	I don't know.
Consultant	Inadequate intake of iron; elderly patients living alone often neglect their food intake, especially if they are short of money also. I don't think that this applies to Mrs N., who in any case is far from what I would regard as elderly. And now I think we should summarize our main conclusions about Mrs N.'s problems based on our analysis of the symptoms in her history.
Consultant	Now, I would like you to present your examination findings (Figure 11.2).
Student	The first thing to note is that Mrs N. is anaemic.
Consultant	Do you think that the anaemia is due to iron deficiency?
Student	I thought we had discussed this earlier. We said it might be an iron-

HISTORY

- Mrs N. has a chronic back problem most likely due to osteo-athritis of the lumbar spine
- her recent and more severe pain in the mid-dorsal region has a different origin and may be due to a neoplastic lesion in the dorsal spine
- the anorexia and loss of weight may also be manifestations of a neoplastic condition
- the excessive fatigue is likely to be due, at least in part, to anaemia: a possible cause of this anaemia may be GI bleeding due to drugs but the other possibility is that it may be caused by neoplasia
- the long-standing smoking raises the possibility of a primary lesion of the lung which might have then secondarily involved the spine
- another possible primary site for a lesion which might then go on to affect the spine is Mrs N.'s uterus
- the recent nocturia may be due to renal failure and if that is the case then the question of myeloma should be considered to account for both the spinal lesion and the renal failure

deficiency anaemia due to blood loss from the gastro-intestinal tract as a result of her tablets.

Consultant	But is Mrs N.'s anaemia due to this cause?
Student	I don't think we can answer that without some investigations.

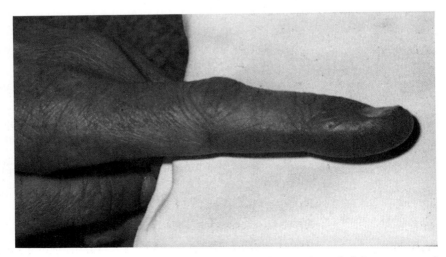

Figure 11.1 Koilonychia in a patient with chronic iron-deficiency anaemia showing the typical 'spoon shape' depression of the finger nails.

Consultant	Isn't there any other way you can tell from your examination?
Student	I don't think so.
Consultant	What about Mrs N.'s finger nails?
Student	I see, you are asking about koilonychia. I didn't look specially for this but I think the finger nails are normal.
Consultant	Koilonychia is a very helpful indication of chronic iron-deficiency anaemia, but it is often forgotten by students in their examination of the patient — do try to remember this sign next time; the nails may not show the classical 'spoon shape' — I've a good picture of this here (Figure 11.1) — but may tend to be just flattened. Angular stomatitis is another sign which has been described in chronic iron-deficiency anaemia, but I have rarely encountered it myself. We mentioned another possible cause of anaemia in a lady of Mrs N.'s age — do you remember what it was?
Student	Pernicious anaemia.
Consultant	Did you find any evidence of this condition in your examination?
Student	I thought you could only diagnose this from the blood count, marrow examination and the serum B_{12} level.
Consultant	You have summarized the investigation of pernicious anaemia admirably, but I wasn't wanting that. What I'm asking you is whether there are any helpful clinical signs that you might find in a patient in whom you suspect pernicious anaemia?
Student	You could get neurological signs like subacute combined degeneration of the spinal cord.
Consultant	And did you look for this?
Student	Not specifically, but I did examine her nervous system and thought it was normal.
Consultant	What neurological signs would you look for if you were suspecting subacute combined degeneration?
Student	You would get a combination of pyramidal signs and posterior column signs.
Consultant	Good, but don't forget signs of peripheral neuritis may be the earliest manifestation of the neurological involvement caused by vitamin B_{12} deficiency. Apart from the neurological complications of pernicious anaemia, is there any other simple sign which might give you a clue?
Student	I can't think of any.
Consultant	Have you looked at Mrs N.'s tongue?
Student	It was normal.
Consultant	Can the tongue help in the diagnosis of anaemia?
Student	You can get glossitis with iron-deficiency anaemia.

Consultant	That's right — the tongue may then be red and sore What about the tongue in pernicious anaemia?
Student	I remember now — you mean she might have an atrophic glossitis?
Consultant	Yes, the tongue is then pale and smooth all over. It's a common sign in pernicious anaemia and you should always consciously look for it. Carry on with your examination.
Student	The pulse and blood pressure were normal and I couldn't find any abnormal signs in the heart.
Consultant	If I were presenting the findings, I would be inclined to mention Mrs N.'s breasts next in relation to suspected mitotic involvement of the spine. You must try to get your priorities in the right order!
Student	I'm very sorry — I forgot to examine her breasts.
Consultant	(To patient) Mrs N., would you mind if the student examines your breasts?
	After the patient says she doesn't mind at all, the student examines Mrs N.'s breasts and pronounces them normal.
Consultant	An essential part of the examination of the breasts is to examine both axillae for glands also, which you did not do — try to remember this for the future. Mrs N. does not have any abnormal axillary glands. Now the next relevant examination to present in Mrs N. is the back rather than the cardiovascular system, since this is more likely to help with the diagnosis.
Student	I couldn't examine her back very well in bed so I asked her to get out of bed and I stood her by the side.
Consultant	That's the right way to examine a patient's back but you must of course make sure that the patient is not in any severe back pain at the time.
Student	I did ask her that before I got her out of bed — she had recently taken her pain-relieving tablet and she said it would be all right for her to get out of bed to allow me to examine her.
Consultant	Tell us your findings.
Student	Her movements were very limited — she could hardly bend forward at all to touch her toes. She said it was very painful.
Consultant	Did you test any other movements?
Student	I had to do it carefully because I didn't want to cause her more discomfort than I had to; I managed to test bending backwards which was also limited and rather painful. I didn't test lateral flexion of the spine because I thought that would be too much of a strain on her spine.
Consultant	You were quite right to be careful and it was very good of Mrs N. to allow you to do what you have. Did you test for any local spinal tenderness?

Student	Yes, I tapped her gently over her spine and she does have two tender spots — one low down in the dorsal spine and the other one higher up but I wasn't sure exactly which vertebrae they were.
Consultant	What do these findings suggest?
Student	That she has probably got some lesions in these vertebrae.
Consultant	What sort of lesions?
Student	I think they are likely to be neoplastic.
Consultant	I agree. Did you check her straight leg raising?
Student	I wasn't sure whether it might be too painful so I didn't do it.
Consultant	Your concern is commendable and I understand your hesitation. It is an important test if you need to decide about root irritation from osteo-arthritis of the lumbar spine or from a prolapsed disc. As we don't think this is the cause of Mrs N.'s current back problem, I agree that we can forgot his test in view of her pain.
	There are of course other less uncomfortable tests which may help in diagnosing root pain, aren't there?
Student	You might get sensory changes in the leg.
Consultant	You can also get changes in the deep reflexes. Did you look for any neurological abnormalities of this type when you examined her nervous system?
Student	As I mentioned earlier, I couldn't find any abnormality in Mrs N.'s nervous system.
Consultant	As long as you kept the possibility of root irritation consciously in your mind when you were making the examination! You should always know exactly what you are looking for whenever you examine a patient, and in this context, let me remind you of a very relevant biblical quotation — do you know what it is?
Student	No, I don't — I'm afraid I have rather neglected my biblical studies lately; perhaps it's because of all this medical stuff I'm expected to learn!
Consultant	Touché! The quotation is: 'Seek and ye shall find'. Try to remember it whenever you examine a patient.
	Before we leave the question of root irritation in the leg, it might be useful to remind ourselves of the nerve roots involved in the knee and ankle jerks.
Student	I think the ankle jerk is S1 and 2, and the knee jerk is L3 and 4.
Consultant	That is correct. To add the sensory changes for completeness, an S1 lesion produces sensory impairment on the sole of the foot, L4 affect the front of the thigh and the medial side of the leg and L5 the lateral side of the leg and the dorsum of the foot.
	Are there any other examination findings that you wish to mention?
Student	Her lungs were clear.

Consultant	What abnormality were you looking for?
Student	For any evidence of a bronchial neoplasm.
Consultant	Yes, that would be very relevant in the light of our earlier discussion about secondary involvement of the spine. What particular lung signs would you have in mind?
Student	Any focal signs such as collapse.
Consultant	You can also find an unresolved pneumonia or pleurisy with or without effusion. It is said in the textbooks that you can find a localized persistent wheeze over a constricted bronchus — I have never come across it. There are of course other important signs of a bronchial neoplasm away from the lungs, aren't there?
Student	There was no finger clubbing and there were no neck glands.
Consultant	Those are two important signs. If you mention glands, though, don't forget axillary glands as well as neck glands. Mrs N. doesn't have any axillary glands — we have checked. There is another important manifestation of involvement of glands in the vicinity of the lungs — do you know what I am getting at?
Student	Do you mean mediastinal obstruction?
Consultant	That's right. Can you suggest any other signs associated with bronchial neoplasm?
Student	It could involve the liver; I could not find an enlarged liver when I examined Mrs N.
Consultant	There are several non-metastatic manifestations — can you name any of them?
Student	You can get a peripheral neuropathy.
Consultant	Anything else?
Student	Cushing's syndrome.
Consultant	Do you know how that is caused?
Student	I think it's due to production of ACTH by the lesion.
Consultant	That's right, especially if the lesion consists of oat cells. Do you know whether any other ectopic hormones can be produced?
Student	I can't think of any others.

Consultant	You can get antidiuretic hormone leading to a syndrome resembling diabetes insipidus.
	    There are other so-called para-neoplastic syndromes including myopathy, syndromes resembling myasthenia gravis and motor neurone disease and thrombophlebitis migrans.
	    Fortunately, Mrs N. has none of these problems.
	    Are there any other examination findings that we ought to know about?

Student	I don't think so.
Consultant	There is one other important organ we should mention in a woman if we are considering a spread of a mitotic lesion.
Student	We've already mentioned the uterus earlier in our discussion, but I haven't done a pelvic examination in Mrs N.
Consultant	That is an examination which is best left to the gynaecologists.

The uterus and the breast are often overlooked in patients presenting as medical problems. It is important never to take it for granted that a problem is a medical one because the patient is referred to a medical clinic, and these two organs are of considerable significance if the problem is likely to have a neoplastic origin.

Now, I think we can summarize the relevant examination findings and what conclusions we draw from them:

EXAMINATION

- we have confirmed the anaemia
- there is no evidence of koilonychia (chronic iron deficiency) or atrophic glossitis (pernicious anaemia) or subacute combined degeneration of the spinal cord (pernicious anaemia)
- she has localized tenderness over two of the dorsal vertebrae, possibly due to neoplasm
- there is limitation of spinal movements but no evidence of root irritation to suggest a prolapsed disc
- there was no evidence of a primary lesion of the breast or lung which might secondarily have involved the spine, and there was no evidence of secondary lesions elsewhere
- a pelvic examination has not been carried out to see if there was any recurrence of the uterine lesion — it was thought that this is best left to a gynaecologist but it should be checked

---

Consultant	Now, I would like you to consider how we should investigate Mrs N.'s problems. What is the first test you would like?
Student	A blood count.
Consultant	Why do you want a blood count?
Student	Because Mrs N. is anaemic and I think it will help to tell us how severe the anaemia is.
Consultant	All right, that's a reasonable request but what you are really asking for is not a 'blood count' but a haemoglobin level and a blood film, which might give you some help in indicating the type of anaemia. Try to be as specific as you can in asking for any test — it's a good mental discipline and an aid to perspicacity.

Here is Mrs N.'s blood count and I am showing you the full blood

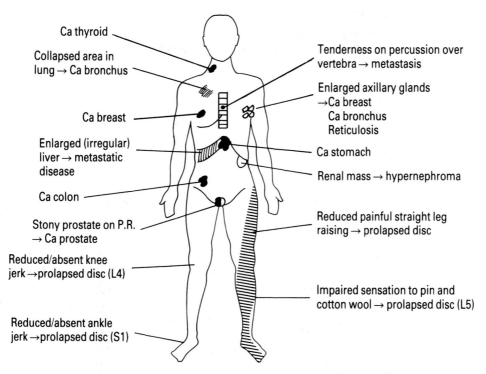

Figure 11.2 Possible signs of diagnostic help in back pain of sudden onset.

count, not just the haemoglobin, since it shows some interesting findings. May we have your comments please?

		Normal range
Haemoglobin	8.7	12–16 g/dl
Red cell count	2.7	$4.0–5.2 \times 10^{12}$/L
Leucocytes	3.5	$4.5–11.0 \times 10^9$/L
Thrombocytes	110	$150–400 \times 10^9$/L

blood film — normocytic normochromic, some plasma cells seen, rouleaux formation

Student	First of all it confirms the anaemia which is not due to iron deficiency.
Consultant	That is correct, so the anaemia is not due to gastro-intestinal blood loss. What do you think of the white cell count and the platelets?
Student	They are both reduced.
Consultant	What is the significance of that?
Student	Does it suggest marrow depression?

Consultant	It's not so much direct marrow depression as the likelihood of marrow infiltration, and you might see with what if you study the report carefully.
Student	By plasma cells.
Consultant	That's right — do you know what this indicates?
Student	This would suggest myelomatosis.
Consultant	What is the significance of the rouleaux formation mentioned in the blood film?
Student	I'm not sure.
Consultant	In myeloma the red cells may become coated with an abnormal immuno-globulin and this causes them to clump together more easily to form rouleaux. What other tests would you like?
Student	An ESR would be an important test since this is always very high in myeloma.
Consultant	Mrs N.'s ESR is 132 mm/hr which confirms what you say. What is the next test?
Student	I think we should X-ray the spine.
Consultant	This is obviously a very important test because of Mrs N.'s back pain. Here are the films if you would like to let us have your comments (Figure 11.3).
Student	There seem to be crush fractures of this lower dorsal vertebra and I think there are also crush fractures in these two vertebrae higher up.
Consultant	Those are good observations and accurate. What do you think is the cause?
Student	The most likely cause is myeloma.
Consultant	I agree with you. We will discuss confirmation of the diagnosis of myeloma shortly, but let me ask you first whether there are any other X-rays you would like to see in Mrs N.?
Student	I think a skull X-ray would be worth doing because the skull is often involved in myeloma.
Consultant	Here is the skull X-ray (Figure 11.4).
Student	There are a lot of translucent areas.
Consultant	What do you think they could be due to?
Student	The most likely cause would be myeloma in the light of our other findings.
Consultant	Could there be any other cause for this appearance?
Student	You can get a similar appearance in mitotic deposits.
Consultant	That is the second important cause of multiple translucent areas in the skull — there is a third cause that you should also think of. Do you know what it is?

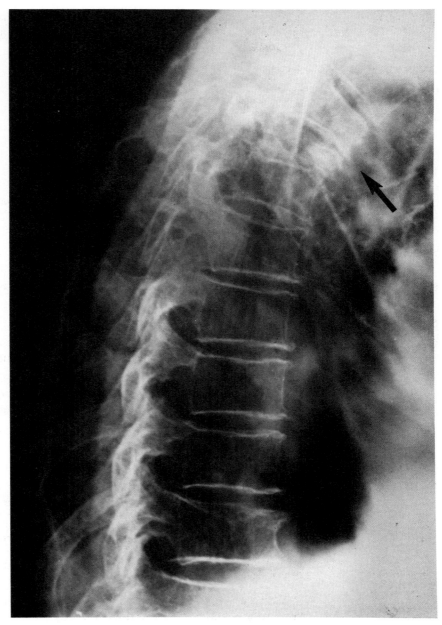

Figure 11.3 X-ray of Mrs N.'s dorsal spine showing myelomatous involvement and crush fractures in the upper dorsal vertebrae (arrowed).

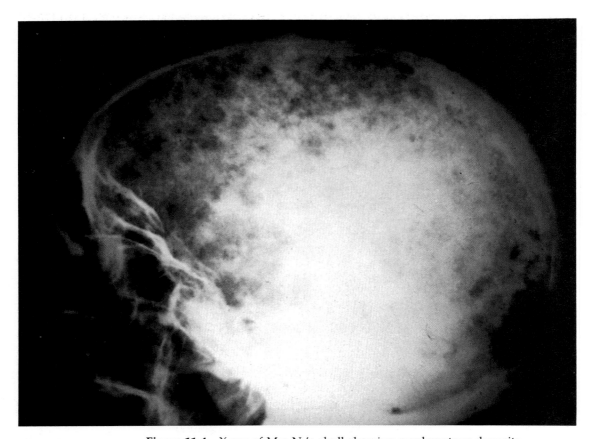

Figure 11.4   X-ray of Mrs N.'s skull showing myelomatous deposits.

Student	I'm sorry.
Consultant	Hyperparathyroidism, which produces what is rather fancifully called a 'pepper pot' appearance in the skull. Here is an example of a 'pepper pot' skull (Figure 11.5). Is there any other X-ray that is useful in diagnosing myeloma?
Consultant	Is there any other X-ray that is useful in diagnosing myeloma?
Student	The pelvis can sometimes be affected.
Consultant	That's right. We have X-rayed Mrs N.'s pelvis and it is normal. Any other X-ray we should do — not necessarily connected with myeloma?
Student	We should X-ray Mrs N.'s chest in view of the other possible diagnosis we discussed — a primary lesion of the lung.
Consultant	Good. Mrs N.'s chest X-ray shows some heavy markings at the lung bases due no doubt to chronic bronchitis from her smoking, but there is no evidence of a lung lesion of the type you mentioned.

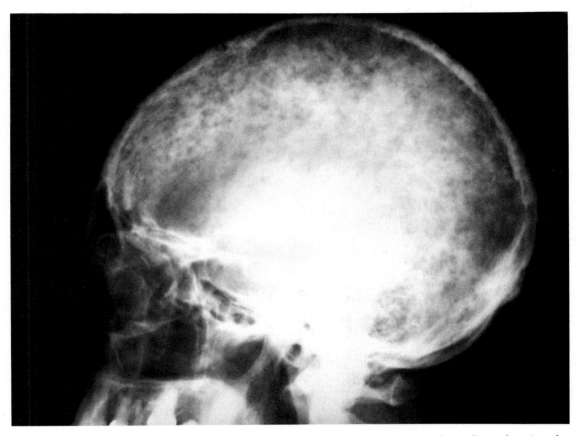

Figure 11.5 Skull X-ray in a patient with hyperparathyroidism showing the typical 'pepper-pot' appearance.

	Now, I think we should get back to confirming the diagnosis of myeloma. How should we do this?
Student	We could examine the urine for Bence Jones* protein.
Consultant	Yes, that is a useful and simple test for myeloma though it is not always present — perhaps in about 50% of patients. Would you know how to do this test yourself?
Student	I'm sorry I don't.
Consultant	When I was a student, we did all the simple urine tests ourselves in our patients and I think it a shame that students do not have the same degree of self-reliance today.

* H. Bence Jones (1814–1873) was a renowned English physician who was also a highly skilled chemist. He was elected FRS and became Secretary of the Royal Institution. He was a friend of Faraday and wrote his biography.

You would heat the urine in a test tube over a Bunsen* burner; Bence Jones protein precipitates out at 60° and then redissolves as you raise the temperature further to boiling point — it will precipitate out again as the urine cools.

Now, what do you think is the really diagnostic test in myeloma?

Student   Electrophoresis of the serum.

Consultant   That's right. We have found an abnormal band in Mrs N. which is consistent with myelomatosis. Immunophoresis has shown us that this abnormal protein is a monoclonal immuno-globulin which is called 'M' protein and is diagnostic of myeloma. It is when this abnormal immuno-globulin spills over into the urine that you find Bence Jones protein.

There is perhaps just one more test we could do that would clinch the diagnosis of myeloma.

Student   You could examine the bone marrow for myeloma cells.

Consultant   That's right and we have found Mrs N.'s marrow infiltrated with a lot of plasma (myeloma) cells, some of which had spilled over into the peripheral blood as we saw in the blood count.

We could perhaps mention one more test which is usually done in myeloma but is non-specific.

OUTCOME

Mrs N.'s bone pain was treated with local irradiation to the dorsal spine with rapid relief of the pain.

She was given a blood transfusion of 4 units which increased the haemoglobin level to 12 g/dl.

The renal failure improved with rehydration and the blood urea fell to 14 mmol/L.

It was decided to give her intermittent chemotherapy with melphalan 10 mg/day for one week together with prednisolone 60 mg/day, and this course was repeated twice more at intervals of 6 weeks. A satisfactory response was shown by clinical improvement and a progressive decrease in the level of the abnormal paraprotein as shown in the 'M' band on electrophoresis.

During subsequent follow-up over a period of 18 months her clinical condition remained satisfactory though she did require one further course of melphalan and prednisolone when the paraprotein level increased again. Renal function remained stable, the haemoglobin level fell only slightly and maintained at around 11 g/dl and there was no recurrence of back pain.

---

* R.W.E. von Bunsen (1811–1899) was Professor of Chemistry at Heidelberg. He introduced spectrum analysis.

Student   I don't know which test you mean.

Consultant   The serum calcium level is often raised, and this is important because it might lead to renal damage. Myelomatous infiltration itself also affects the kidney and can cause renal failure; you will remember that we thought Mrs N.'s nocturia might be a manifestation of this and her blood urea level has confirmed this diagnosis — it was raised to 23 mmol/L (normal 3.6–7.0 mmol/L).

LEARNING POINTS

Organic causes of weight loss

- endocrine
    diabetes mellitus
    thyrotoxicosis
    Addison's disease
- chronic infection
    tuberculosis
    infective endocarditis
    brucellosis
    fungal infection
- gastro-intestinal
    inflammatory bowel disease
    ulcerative colitis
    Crohn's disease
    malabsorption
    chronic pancreatitis
    peptic ulcer
- malignancy
    carcinoma
    myeloma
    reticulosis
- uraemia

Causes of chronic back pain

- osteo-arthritis of the spine
- prolapsed intervertebral disc
- ankylosing spondylitis
- tuberculosis of the spine
- congenital e.g. spondylolisthesis
- psychogenic

Causes of very high ESR (>100 mm/hr)

- carcinomatosis
- myelomatosis
- temporal arteritis
- polymyalgia rheumatica
- collagen disease e.g. SLE
- infection
    pulmonary
    urinary tract

Symptoms of myelomatosis

- loss of weight
- bone pain

- susceptibility to infection (impaired immunological response)
- renal pain due to stone (hypercalcaemia)
- symptoms of renal failure

Causes of anaemia in myeloma

- bone marrow infiltration
- haemolysis
- renal failure
- associated infections

Diagnostic tests in myeloma

- blood count
  anaemia
  leucopenia
  thrombocytopenia
  rouleaux
  plasma cells (occasionally)
- ESR > 100 mm/hr
- bone marrow
  infiltration with plasma cells
- urine
  Bence Jones protein (50%)
- biochemical
  hypercalcaemia
  uraemia
- X-rays
  spine, skull and pelvis —
    osteolytic lesions
    pathological fractures
- immunology
  electrophoresis — abnormal 'M' band
  immunophoresis — monoclonal immuno-globulin

Causes of osteolytic lesions in the skull X-ray

- carcinomatosis
- myelomatosis
- hyperparathyroidism

12

Polyarthritis

Student Mrs S.S. is a 44-year-old housewife who has been admitted for treatment of her arthritis.

She gives a 10-year history of arthritis which is slowly getting worse. At first the arthritis affected just her hands but it has gradually spread to involve her wrists, elbows, knees and even her neck. She has been treated with a variety of drugs some of which had upset her stomach so she had to stop taking them. For the last three years or so she has been taking prednisolone. She has also had a lot of physiotherapy which helped but only temporarily while she was on treatment.

The problem that has brought her into hospital now is that her knees have been very bad, particularly the left knee. The knees became bad about six weeks ago, and she had injections into both knees about three weeks ago: although the right knee has settled, the left seems to be getting worse — in fact she had so much pain in the knee that her GP has admitted her as an emergency. As far as the other joints are concerned, her wrists and fingers have also been very painful over the last few weeks and her dose of prednisolone has been increased from 2 tablets a day to 3 tablets a day over the last two weeks which has helped her hands, but she thinks that her left knee has become worse.

In the past history, she had an attack of pleurisy about one month ago which she says has left her with an irritating cough, and she thinks she is more breathless than usual since the attack.

The family history is interesting because her mother has suffered from arthritis for many years. She also has one sister who has trouble with her bowels.

Mrs S. does not smoke and only drinks on special occasions. The treatment she is having at present is 3 tablets of prednisolone a day and she also uses a lot of paracetamol.

Consultant The problem that we have to deal with is arthritis. Could you let us know what you think about this?

Student I thought that the history sounded like rheumatoid arthritis.

Consultant That's a sensible suggestion. What do you base this diagnosis on?

Student	She has a long history of recurrent episodes of arthritis mainly affecting the smaller joints, and her mother has a similar complaint.
Consultant	Those are two good points. You quite rightly mentioned her small joints but what about her neck — didn't you say that her neck was troubling her also?
Student	I think that RA can affect the neck.
Consultant	Yes, that can occur, and it has been claimed that as many as 80% of patients with RA have neck involvement. It is important to distinguish it from cervical spondylosis which is also very common — the distinction is made on the basis of the radiological changes in the neck.
	What other possibilities should we consider in the differential diagnosis of chronic polyarthritis?
Student	I suppose I should mention osteo-arthritis.
Consultant	Yes, osteo-arthritis ought to be considered. Traditionally, it used to be regarded as purely a degenerative condition affecting the larger joints, but research has shown that it has a multifactorial origin, including genetic, metabolic and probably inflammatory factors in the causation.
	Although it affects the larger joints, it can also involve the small joints — do you know which ones particularly?
Student	No, I'm sorry, I don't know.
Consultant	It often affects the terminal inter-phalangeal joints of the fingers, especially in older people: this produces a very distinctive sign — do you know what it is called?

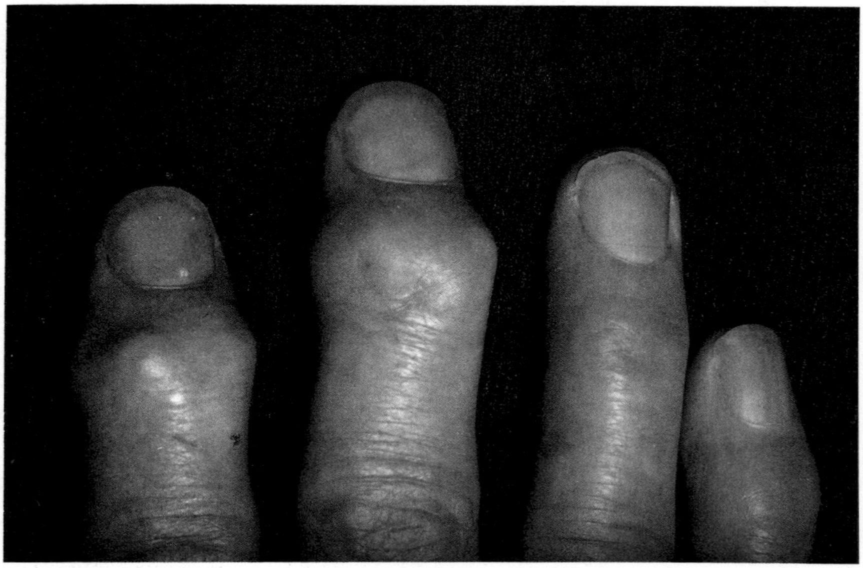

Figure 12.1 Heberden's nodes.

Student	No.
Consultant	It produces Heberden's nodes. Who was Heberden?
Student	I think he was a famous physician in the last century.
Consultant	William Heberden (1710–1801) was an eminent London physician, a Fellow of the Royal Society and also a leading Latin and Hebrew scholar. He gave a classic description of angina which has never been bettered, as well as writing expertly about chicken-pox and night-blindness.
Student	Can I ask you about something which has confused me in the past? Sometimes my teachers have talked about osteo-arthritis and sometimes they call it osteo-arthrosis. I've always thought the two conditions were the same — am I right?
Consultant	I can understand your confusion — osteo-arthritis and osteo-arthrosis are terms which are often used indiscriminately. I think it may be a reflection of the traditional view that the condition is purely a degenerative one and therefore shouldn't be called arthritis but arthrosis. As I mentioned earlier, this view is wrong, so osteo-arthritis is perfectly correct.
	It is probably better to restrict the term osteo-arthrosis to those conditions in which damage occurs to joints as a result of occupational trauma, like heavy manual work affecting the spine, hips and knees, and the use of vibratory tools affecting the elbows and wrist joints.
	What other inflammatory causes of polyarthritis should we be considering?
Student	What about gout?
Consultant	Does gout usually cause polyarthritis?
Student	No, not usually, but I think it can sometimes.
Consultant	You're quite right — it can affect multiple joints, which is perhaps not appreciated as widely as it should, but it is rare in polyarthritic form. It is also rare in females. There is a particular sign which you should look for in chronic gout, but we'll leave that till you present your examination findings.
	Gout is possible in Mrs S. but unlikely.
	Any other conditions?
Student	Collagen disease is another possibility.
Consultant	Which collagen disease did you have in mind?
Student	Systemic lupus erythematosus.
Consultant	Yes, I agree that diagnosis should be considered. Is there anything else in the history to support SLE?
Student	You can get pleurisy in SLE and Mrs S. did have pleurisy a few months ago.
Consultant	Pleurisy is common in SLE but it can also occur in RA. What other symptoms might you get in SLE?

Student	I believe that the kidneys can be involved.
Consultant	SLE does lead sometimes to glomerulo-nephritis which is unlikely to produce much in the way of symptoms but does show relevant signs which we won't pursue until we come to your examination.
	Do you know any other features of SLE?
Student	I can't think of any.
Consultant	A 'butterfly' rash and skin photosensitivity are among the commonest manifestations. Other less common features include symptoms such as paraesthesiae or muscle weakness due to peripheral neuritis, chest pain due to pericarditis, breathlessness and ankle swelling due to myocarditis and lumps in the neck, axillae or groins due to lymphadenopathy.
	Apart from pleurisy, Mrs S. doesn't have any other manifestations of SLE, but obviously we must keep this diagnosis in mind and re-assess it when we examine Mrs S. and investigate her later. We mustn't forget also that polyarthritis can occur in other types of collagen disease such as polyarteritis, systemic sclerosis or mixed connective tissue disease, but it is less common than in SLE.
	To return to the arthritis of SLE, is there any way you might be able to distinguish it from that of RA? What about the joint pains in the two conditions?
Student	I thought they were similar in that they both affect the small joints.
Consultant	That is not what I meant. The joint pains differ in that the pain is constant in RA unlike SLE where the pain flits from joint to joint — like rheumatic fever.
	What about the joints themselves — do they differ in the two conditions? It might help your answer if I said that SLE causes arthralgia rather than arthritis.
Student	This would mean that the joints are unlikely to be as swollen and as inflamed as in RA.
Consultant	That's right. Another important distinguishing point is that the joints are symmetricially involved in RA, whereas in SLE joint involvement tends to be asymmetrical.
	There is one other very distinctive symptom in RA joints, apart from pain, which you won't find in SLE. Do you know what this is?
Student	Yes, I think so — morning stiffness, but I forgot to ask Mrs S. about this.
Consultant	This is an important question you must always ask when you are considering a diagnosis of RA.
	Would you like to ask her now?
Student	Mrs S., can you tell me if your joints feel stiff when you first wake up in the morning?
Patient	That is one of my main problems. I can hardly move my fingers in the morning and it takes a few hours before I can get my hands moving properly.

Consultant	That is very suggestive of RA.
	Let us return to the differential diagnosis of chronic polyarthritis — have you any other suggestions to make?
Student	Can you give me any clues?
Consultant	Why not? I feel in a helpful mood today. Is there any skin disorder that you know of that may be associated with joint problems?
Student	Oh yes, psoriasis.
Consultant	Good. Do you know what joints are usually affected in psoriatic arthropathy?
Student	Yes, I can remember that — it is the terminal joints of the fingers.
Consultant	That's right — the terminal inter-phalangeal joints of the fingers; other joints are very rarely affected. There is a distinctive sign that often goes with this joint involvement but I think we will leave this until you come to your examination findings. The absence of skin manifestations of psoriasis in Mrs S. would make psoriatic arthropathy less likely, though sometimes psoriatic arthropathy develops before the skin lesions.
	To help you further in your quest for other causes of polyarthritis, can I suggest you might turn your attention to Mrs S.'s nether regions or is that clue too subtle for you?
Student	I'm not too sure what you are getting at.
Consultant	Then it's just as well you don't have to pass a motion on it.
	Laughter all round.
Student	That's not bad — I like it! Thank you for the clue. You obviously mean ulcerative colitis.
Consultant	And Crohn's* disease also — we group the two conditions together and call them inflammatory bowel disease, or, perhaps more pedantically, enteropathic arthritis. They are often very difficult to distinguish even after detailed investigation. Apart from diarrhoea, do you know any other distinctive symptoms of these conditons?
Student	Obviously arthritis is one of them.
Consultant	Any others?
Student	I think you can get skin rashes.
Consultant	This occurs more often with ulcerative colitis than with Crohn's disease. Do you know what type of rash?
Student	I remember pyoderma gangrenosum.
Consultant	Yes, that's the classical one in the textbooks — I have never seen it

* B.B. Crohn was an American physician who first described his disease in 1932 when he was President of the American Gastro-enterology Society.

	myself. A more frequent rash in my experience is erythema nodosum. Any other symptoms?
Student	You can get involvement of the spine.
Consultant	Yes, ankylosing spondylitis may occur — this is commoner in Crohn's disease.
	Have you shot your bolt now or can you think of any other manifestations?
Student	I can't think of any others at the moment.
Consultant	The other symptoms which may sometimes occur are painful eyes, due to uveitis or episcleritis, a sore mouth due to aphthous ulceration, and liver involvement leading to symptoms of hepatitis or cholangitis.
	Mrs S. has none of these manifestations so I think we can forget about inflammatory bowel disease.
	Do you have any other suggestions for the differential diagnosis of chronic polyarthritis?
Student	I think I've reached the end of my differential diagnosis.
Consultant	There is one cause which is always worth considering, though I don't think you'll come across it very often, Reiter's* disease. Do you know anything about this condition?
Student	I think that you get urethritis as well as polyarthritis.
Consultant	That's right — and the third component of the triad of features which makes up the syndrome of Reiter's disease is conjunctivitis. It usually presents as an acute syndrome but it may occasionally follow a chronic course. The cause is unknown but it can be transmitted sexually. Since Mrs S. has neither urethritis nor conjunctivitis I think we can forget about Reiter's disease.
	There are of course other sexually-transmitted diseases which may manifest in arthritis. Do you know what these are?
Student	Gonorrhoea can cause arthritis.
Consultant	It is usually associated with a mono-articular type of arthritis rather than a polyarthritis, and the other condition worth keeping in mind is infection with chlamydia.
	There are one or two other rare causes of polyarthritis which it might be worth mentioning to finish off the differential diagnosis like amyloidosis, sarcoidosis and malignancy.
	Now, I would like to turn to another important aspect of Mrs S.'s history — the fact that her left knee has not responded adequately to the injection of steroid into the joint and has indeed got worse. Does this suggest anything to you?

* H.C. Reiter (1881–1969) described his syndrome while he was an army doctor with the Hungarian army on the Balkan Front in 1916 (it was actually described first almost 100 years earlier by Sir Benjamin Brodie).

Student	Only that Mrs S. has a severe exacerbation of her arthritis and probably needs more treatment, perhaps by increasing her dose of oral prednisolone.
Consultant	Is there any other possible explanation? Let me give you a clue — it could be related to an adverse side-effect of the cortisone used in the injection.
Student	I don't know of any harmful effect of intra-articular cortisone.
Consultant	It's not a direct effect of the drug itself, but it can encourage or facilitate another adverse event in the joint.
Student	You mean infection?
Consultant	Exactly! I'm sure that you know steroids encourage the spread of infection anywhere in the body by suppressing the inflammatory response. If it happens in the knee then you may get a septic arthritis or pyoarthrosis. This is a very serious complication and we must make sure we don't miss it, especially as patients with RA are much more prone to infection anyway.
	Would you like to comment at this point on the relevance of Mrs S.'s family history?
Student	I've already mentioned her mother's arthritis as a factor in favour of Mrs S. having RA because it runs in families.
Consultant	What about the sister and her bowel problem?
Student	I suppose this could also be relevant if the sister had ulcerative colitis or Crohn's disease — we mentioned previously the relationship with arthritis.
Consultant	Inflammatory bowel disease and RA are both considered to be auto-immune diseases and so may well coexist. Do you know of any other auto-immune diseases which may coexist and run in families?
Student	Diabetes is thought to be an auto-immune disease.
Consultant	Any others?
Student	Thyroid disease, I think.
Consultant	Do you know what kind of thyroid disease?
Student	Myxoedema.
Consultant	To be more accurate, what you're thinking of is Hashimoto's* thyroiditis; although it often leads to myxoedema — some experts say always — it may also present occasionally with thyrotoxicosis.
	The other two auto-immune conditions to mention are pernicious anaemia and hypoparathyroidism.
	At this point I think that we have got as much out of the history as we can so I suggest that we summarize our conclusions:

* H. Hashimoto (1881–1934) was a Japanese surgeon who wrote his MD Thesis on 'Struma Lymphomatosa' (thyroiditis).

> HISTORY
>
> - the long history of recurrent polyarthritis affecting the smaller joints suggests RA
> - the family history of arthritis and chronic bowel trouble suggests an inherited predisposition to auto-immune disease
> - the recent deterioration of the left knee after an intra-articular injection of cortisone raises the possibility of septic arthritis
> - the past history of pleurisy may be associated with RA, but the alternative diagnosis of SLE should also be kept in mind

Consultant   Now, I would like to turn to your examination findings and can I suggest that you focus your attention first on the polyarthritis.

Student   The main joints affected are the hands and the knees.

There is ulnar deviation of the right hand with redness and swelling over the metacarpo-phalangeal joints in both hands, but more marked on the right. Mrs S. found it painful to grip my fingers with either hand.

Both wrists are swollen with limited movement and some pain on movement.

Both knees are swollen, especially on the left, which is red and tender — I couldn't really examine this knee properly because it was so painful to touch and move, but I did just wonder if there could be some fluid in the joint.

I couldn't find much wrong with the other joints such as the elbows, ankles and the feet.

Consultant   What do these findings suggest?

Student   The involvement of the small joints is very much in favour of RA.

Consultant   Could the joint changes be caused by SLE?

Student   No, I don't think so because we said earlier that SLE does not usually cause much inflammation or swelling.

Consultant   That's right, unless it is assoicated with Jaccoud's* arthritis which can cause permanent stiffness and deformity in the metacarpo-phalangeal joints: incidentally Jaccoud's arthritis can also occur following recurrent rheumatic fever.

We'll come back to SLE in a moment.

To return to the clinical findings, did you examine Mrs S.'s neck?

Student   Yes, and she does have some pain and limitation of movement, particularly when I tilted her head to the left.

Consultant   And what do you think this means?

Student   It could be due to RA affecting her neck joints.

---

* S. Jaccoud (1830–1913) was Professor of Pathology in Paris.

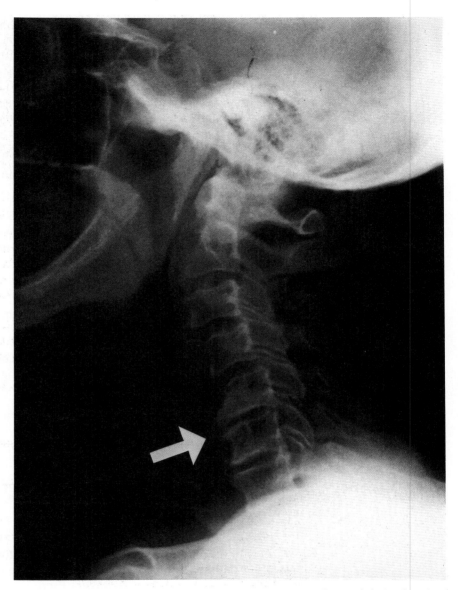

Figure 12.2 Lateral X-ray of the cervical spine in cervical spondylosis showing narrowed disc spaces (arrowed) and the typical lipping (arrowed) in this condition.

Consultant	It could, or it may be due to associated cervical spondylosis (Figure 12.2). What do you make of the findings in her knees?
Student	They are both involved in an acute flare-up of the arthritis and the left one seems more affected than the right.

Consultant	RA usually affects joints symmetrically. The fact that the left knee is a lot worse than the right, and is also so swollen, tender and hot should lead you to suspect a pyo-arthrosis. You will see that she has a high swinging temperature which would be consistent with a septic arthritis — the temperature in RA is not usually so high.
	Now if you were considering SLE, what other signs would you be looking for? First of all what about the joints — would they be any different to RA?
Student	As we said earlier, the joints would be less swollen and inflamed.
Consultant	That's right. Is there any other difference in the joints?
Student	Not that I am aware of.
Consultant	There is much less joint damage in SLE, unless there is associated Jaccoud's arthritis.
	Mrs S.'s joints are deformed which therefore is more suggestive of RA than SLE.
	What other signs would you expect in SLE?
Student	You can get a 'butterfly rash' on the face.
Consultant	That is so — again, this is not present in Mrs S. What else?
Student	The spleen can be enlarged.
Consultant	This can happen in RA also, especially in a particular type of RA associated with abnormalities in the blood picture. What am I referring to?
Student	Felty's* syndrome.
Consultant	That's right — does Mrs S. have an enlarged spleen?
Student	I couldn't feel her spleen.
Consultant	Can you think of any other findings in SLE?
Student	I think you can get a peripheral neuritis.
Consultant	You can in fact get this in all the collagen disorders, including RA, but in my experience it is very rare. Anything else?
Student	I can't think of any more signs.
Consultant	Vasculitis is an important feature of SLE but this too can occur in RA also: you get painful, tender, red spots often in the fingers. Mrs S. has none of these. Talking about the fingers there is one other important sign of SLE — do you know what it is?
Student	Sorry, I don't.
Consultant	You get peri-ungual erythema.
	What about the lymph glands in SLE?
Student	I forgot about these — they can be enlarged.

* A.R. Felty (1895–1964) was an American physician who worked at the Johns Hopkins Medical School and described his syndrome in 1923.

Consultant	That's right, particularly the neck glands, so you should always palpate the neck carefully in a young lady with suspected RA, especially if there are any unusual features.
	Now, I'd like to come back to the rest of your examination findings. Is there anything you want to tell us about the cardiovascular or respiratory systems? (Figure 12.3).
Student	The pulse was 108 and regular, the blood pressure was 145/85, the heart sounds were normal and I couldn't hear any murmurs.
Consultant	Would you expect to hear any murmurs in RA?
Student	I don't think so.
Consultant	You can occasionally get aortic incompetence which is thought to be causally related to the RA. What if the diagnosis was SLE — would you expect any cardiac abnormality?
Student	Yes, I think that you can get involvement of the heart valves in SLE.
Consultant	Do you know what the condition is called?
Student	Yes, I do in fact remember this one; it's called Libman–Sacks syndrome.
Consultant	Well done! I don't suppose you know who Libman–Sacks was, or is it Libman and Sacks?
Student	I'm afraid I don't know.
Consultant	E. Libman (1872–1946) was an American physician working at the famous Mount Sinai Hospital in New York, and B. Sacks (1873–1939) was his pupil.
	Were there any abnormal findings in the lungs?
Student	No, I didn't think so.
Consultant	Can you get any abnormality in the lungs in RA?
Student	You can develop fibrous nodules.
Consultant	It is more correct to call them rheumatoid nodules than fibrous nodules, though they do tend to heal by fibrosis.
	Do you know what this condition is called?
Student	Caplan's* syndrome.
Consultant	Good. Caplan's syndrome is a progressive fibrosis in the lungs, manifesting initially as nodules, developing in the lungs of coalminers with RA. Caplan described the condition when he worked among the Welsh miners. You can also get these rheumatoid nodules occurring in isolation in the lungs and not associated with pneumoconiosis.
	There are other types of pulmonary involvement in RA such as pleurisy with or without effusion; also you can get fibrosing alveolitis.
	Pleural effusions can also occur in SLE.
	To finish the examination, I'll just ask you about the nervous system.

* A. Caplan, a contemporary British physician, born in 1931.

Student	The nervous system seemed normal.
Consultant	Would you expect to find any abnormality in Mrs S.?
Student	Can you get peripheral neuritis with RA?
Consultant	It's written in the books so it must be true! In practice I think it must be rare because I have never seen it myself although I have seen many patients with RA. What I have seen occasionally in rheumatoid arthritis is upper motor neurone involvement due to subluxation in the cervical spine.

The time has come for us to summarize our findings and their significance:

> EXAMINATION
>
> - there is evidence of involvement of the small joints of the hands which suggests rheumatoid arthritis
> - the presence of marked joint swelling and deformity makes it very unlikely that Mrs S. has SLE
> - the hot, red, tender, swollen left knee suggests the likelihood of a septic arthritis
> - there was no evidence of any systemic complication of RA like vasculitis, neuritis or pulmonary involvement
> - Mrs S. also has evidence of cervical spondylosis, though it is possible that the neck changes could be due to RA.

Consultant	Now I think we should discuss investigations. What tests do you think might be helpful in Mrs S.?
Student	First of all, I'd like to do a blood count and ESR.
Consultant	Yes, I agree. What would you be looking for?
Student	The white blood count is likely to be high.
Consultant	Would that be helpful?
Student	It would confirm acute inflammation of the joints due to RA.
Consultant	It might do that but you have already decided that on your clinical findings. If it were very high, however, it would be more useful because it would support the diagnosis of a septic arthritis. What else might be useful in the blood count?
Student	It could show anaemia.
Consultant	Yes, anaemia is common in RA. What is it due to?
Student	Any chronic inflammation like RA can produce anaemia.
Consultant	That is probably the commonest cause of anaemia in RA. What type of anaemia would it be?
Student	I think it would be a normocytic anaemia.

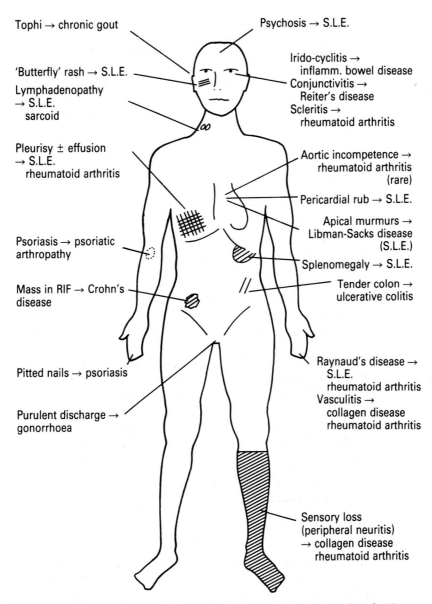

Tophi → chronic gout

'Butterfly' rash → S.L.E.

Lymphadenopathy
→ S.L.E.
   sarcoid

Pleurisy ± effusion
→ S.L.E.
   rheumatoid arthritis

Psoriasis → psoriatic
arthropathy

Mass in RIF → Crohn's
disease

Pitted nails → psoriasis

Purulent discharge →
gonorrhoea

Psychosis → S.L.E.

Irido-cyclitis →
   inflamm. bowel disease
Conjunctivitis →
   Reiter's disease
Scleritis →
   rheumatoid arthritis

Aortic incompetence →
   rheumatoid arthritis
                    (rare)
Pericardial rub → S.L.E.

Apical murmurs →
Libman-Sacks disease
                (S.L.E.)
Splenomegaly → S.L.E.

Tender colon →
   ulcerative colitis

Raynaud's disease →
   S.L.E.
   rheumatoid arthritis
Vasculitis →
   collagen disease
   rheumatoid arthritis

Sensory loss
(peripheral neuritis)
→ collagen disease
   rheumatoid arthritis

Figure 12.3 Possible signs of diagnostic help in polyarthritis.

Consultant	That's right. Any other type of anaemia in RA?
Student	You could get an iron-deficiency anaemia.
Consultant	And what would cause that?
Student	The most likely cause is bleeding from the gastrointestinal tract, and

| | Consultant | this is often caused by the drugs used in treating RA, like aspirin or the non-steroidal anti-inflammatory drugs. |

Consultant   Here is Mrs S.'s blood count. What does it show?

	Mrs S.	Normal range
Haemoglobin	9.9	11.5–16.5 g/dl
White count	21.6	$4.0–11.0 \times 10^9$/L
neutrophil	90%	40–75%
lymphocyte	5%	20–45%
others	5%	

Blood film — microcytosis
                 hypochromia

Student   It shows iron-deficiency anaemia.

Consultant   What do you think is the cause?

Student   It could be due to blood loss from the various drugs she has had for the arthritis.

Consultant   That is the most likely cause.
       What about the white count?

Student   It shows a very high white count, almost all neutrophils, and this could be due to the pyo-arthrosis in the left knee, as you suggested earlier.

Consultant   I would agree. Now you also mentioned the ESR. In what way would this help us in Mrs S.'s problem?

Student   It would be an important pointer to the activity of the RA.

Consultant   That's right — the ESR is a much more useful test in RA than the white count.
       Mrs S.'s ESR is 104 mm/hr.

Student   That is very high; it must indicate active disease.

Consultant   No, I don't think so. I think that it is likely to be so high because of the pus in Mrs S.'s left knee.
       Are there any other tests you think we should do?

Student   We can do a blood test for rheumatoid factor.

Consultant   I think that there is another simpler test we can do before we get on to the more elaborate tests like rheumatoid factor.

Student   We could X-ray her hands.

Consultant   That's more like it. What would you expect to see in RA?

Student   You get destruction of the joint surfaces.

Consultant   That would only occur in advanced cases. What would be the early changes?

Student	I think you get osteoporosis.
Consultant	Yes, that is one of the earliest changes and it occurs in the juxta-articular area. Do you know any other distinctive X-ray changes of RA?
Student	No, I can't think of any.
Consultant	A very distinctive finding which should always make you think of RA is the presence of cystic areas in the bone; they occur just below the articular surfaces of the joints and sometimes also right at the joint margins. In the hands, the changes involve typically the metacarpophalangeal and proximal interphalangeal joints.
	Let me show you Mrs S.'s hand X-rays (Figure 12.4) — you can see the osteoporosis adjacent to the joints, and I think you can also see some small cystic areas as well; these are classical changes of rheumatoid arthritis. The X-ray of Mrs S.'s knee joint didn't show any gross joint destruction but was suspicious of septic infection by showing periostitis.
	The most useful test for diagnosing septic arthritis, however, is . . .?
Student	Is it by blood culture?
Consultant	That is quite a helpful test but is non-specific. The best test is by aspiration and analysis of the synovial fluid. I don't suppose you would know the findings in septic arthritis.
Student	I'm afraid not though if I were to guess I would say that there would be a lot of pus cells.
Consultant	That's a good guess and exactly what does occur. You would get a white cell count of at least 100 000/mm^3 of which at least 75% would be neutrophils; the other biochemical abnormalities in the synovial fluid would be a glucose concentration ratio of fluid/blood of less than 0.5, a high lactic acid concentration and a normal complement level: the other important diagnostic point in the fluid is of course that you will usually be able to culture the organism.
	Examination of the fluid in Mrs S.'s left knee joint showed a white cell count of 130 000/mm^3 with 90% neutrophils and a synovial fluid/blood glucose ratio of only 0.25; we have also cultured a *Staphylococcus aureus* from the fluid.
	Now, if you like, we can return to your rheumatoid factor test. Is it always positive in RA?
Student	I believe so if the disease is active.
Consultant	In fact rheumatoid factor is positive in only 80% of patients with RA so a negative test does not necessarily exclude the condition. Do you want any other tests?
Student	I can't think of any.
Consultant	There is one more test we ought to do to make sure that our diagnosis of rheumatoid is the correct one and we are not in fact dealing with SLE. Do you know what this is?
Student	Is it a collagen screen?

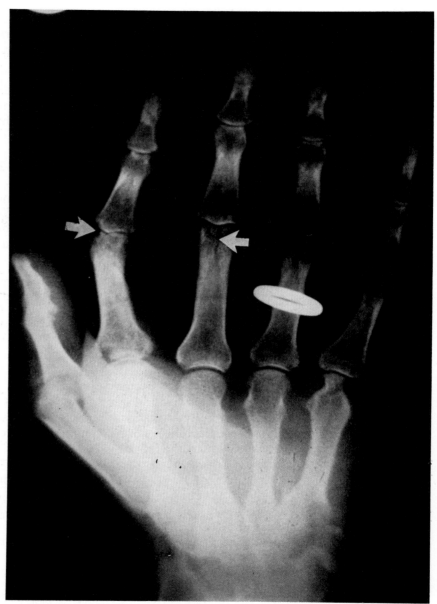

Figure 12.4 X-ray of the hands in chronic rheumatoid arthritis showing the typical juxta-articular osteoporosis (arrowed) and cystic erosions (arrowed).

Consultant	What would you expect to find in SLE?
Student	A positive LE cell test.
Consultant	This test has been largely replaced by the tests for antibodies, the most important of which is antibodies to double-stranded DNA (deoxyribonucleic acid) which is virtually always present in SLE.
	Mrs S.'s test was negative.
	Now, I would like to leave investigation of Mrs S. and spend the last few minutes of this round discussing the treatment of RA. Have you any suggestions?
Student	Non-steroidal anti-inflammatory drugs (NSAIDs) are the usual treatment for RA.
Consultant	Yes, they are, but I think it might be more helpful to have a structured approach to treatment. What is the first requirement for an acute flare-up of RA?
Student	The patient should rest in bed.
Consultant	That's right and more important, the joints should be rested — if necessary by splinting. The physiotherapist can also help a lot with various types of physical treatment including heat, wax baths for stiffness of the joints and exercises to maintain muscle tone around the joints as soon as the acute phase has subsided.
	What drug would you use in this acute phase?
Student	The drug of choice is aspirin.
Consultant	That used to be true but the first choice now is one of the non-steroidal anti-inflammatory drugs which are regarded currently as first-line treatment in rheumatoid arthritis.
	Do you know how aspirin and the NSAIDs work in RA?
Student	I think it has something to do with the prostaglandins.
Consultant	That's right, the drugs inhibit the formation of endogenous prostaglandins which cause inflammation and pain in the joints.
	What about treatment of the RA when the acute phase has subsided?
Student	You can continue with the NSAIDs.
Consultant	I would think that is the usual long-term treatment, but these drugs may have their problems with side-effects; can you tell us about these?
Student	They can irritate the stomach and may cause gastro-intestinal bleeding with the development of anaemia, just as in Mrs S.'s case.
Consultant	Yes, that is a common side-effect. Any others?
Student	You can get oedema of the legs with some of them.
Consultant	Probably to a greater or lesser extent with all of them. Do you know what causes that?
Student	I think it's due to sodium retention.

Consultant	That's right. Let me ask you something else about leg oedema in a patient with RA — is there any other cause that you would think of apart from sodium retention?
Student	It could be due to heart failure.
Consultant	It could but that would be an associated condition and not directly related to the RA.
Student	The other cause which would occur to me would be deep vein thrombosis.
Consultant	It would have to be bilateral to cause oedema in both feet which is very unlikely.
Student	I can't think of any other cause.
Consultant	Amyloidosis is often forgotten. You perhaps didn't know that the commonest cause of amyloidosis in the UK is in fact RA. I've made the diagnosis in several cases myself and it always impresses the audience!
	Let's go back to the clinical manifestations of sodium retention. Can you think of any others apart from oedema?
Student	It can put up the blood pressure.
Consultant	That is why it is important to check the blood pressure regularly in any patient on a NSAID. The other important adverse effect, especially in older patients, is heart failure.
	Now, let's consider what we should do if the NSAIDs are ineffective. Are there any other drugs which might help?
Student	I think you would then consider the use of steroids.
Consultant	Steroids can certainly be very effective in resistant RA but you must be very careful before starting this type of treatment in RA because it may be very difficult to stop. There are some serious hazards to steroid treatment, especially long-term, are there not?
Student	You get gastric irritation and fluid retention just as you do with the NSAIDs.
Consultant	That's correct. Any others?
Student	Long-term steroids can cause osteoporosis.
Consultant	That can be a serious side-effect particularly in elderly patients who may well end up with a fracture as a result, especially in the spine.
Student	I've also seen one or two patients end up with Cushing's syndrome as a result of long-term steroids in RA.
Consultant	That is quite common also with large doses over a prolonged period, say after a few years. Although there is no completely safe upper limit of prednisolone dose for long-term use in rheumatoid arthritis, do you know what is generally regarded as an acceptable dose?
ent	I would think about 10 mg/day.

Consultant	I would put it a bit lower — say 7.5 mg/day, or if feasible even lower still at 5.0 mg/day. Are there any other side-effects that you can think of?
Student	Diabetes can occur.
Consultant	That may be part of a Cushingoid syndrome or it may occur as a separate condition on its own. While we're on biochemical matters, is there any special biochemical measurement that we should keep in mind when we are treating a patient with high dose or long-term steroids?
Student	Do you mean apart from the sugar to see if they have developed diabetes?
Consultant	I wasn't referring to the blood sugar.
Student	The serum potassium level is important because the steroid can cause loss of potassium through the kidneys.
Consultant	Why is hypokalaemia so important, especially in patients with RA who may be in heart failure?
Student	It can lead to cardiac arrhythmias.
Consultant	Especially if the patient was having digoxin for the heart failure. Are there any other types of drug treatment available apart from steroids?
Student	The other two drugs available in resistant RA are gold and penicillamine.
Consultant	Well done. You seem to have a good knowledge of the management of RA.
Student	I have just finished a rheumatology appointment.
Consultant	That explains it! Gold and penicillamine are useful second-line drugs but they do have some drawbacks. Can you remind us of some of the side-effects?
Student	Well, both of the drugs can produce rashes and also depress the bone marrow leading to pancytopenia.
Consultant	Thrombocytopenia is usually the first manifestation of bone-marrow suppression, though it may go on to pancytopenia. Is there any other important renal complication?
Student	Yes, they can also cause nephrotic syndrome.
Consultant	The other side-effects that are worth mentioning with both drugs are mouth ulcers and gastro-intestinal upsets. Can you think of any other drugs for RA?
Student	The only other one that occurs to me, which I saw used when I was doing rheumatology was chloroquine.
Consultant	Chloroquine is primarily an anti-malarial drug but it has been found useful in some cases of RA. Do you know the main hazard with this drug?
Student	It can cause damage to the retina.

Consultant	That's right, so patients on this treatment should have a regular ophthalmic check every 6 months or so. There is a closely related drug, hydroxychloroquine, which is less likely to produce retinal damage so this is the better drug to use.
	Sulphasalazine is another drug which has been found to be of value in treatment of RA and can now be considered as a standard second-line drug.
	There is one other type of drug worth mentioning in resistant RA — do you know which?
Student	No, I am afraid you have got me on this one.
Consultant	In severe progressive and unresponsive RA, especially with serious extra-articular manifestations, immunotherapy with drugs like azathioprine or cyclophosphamide can be tried.
	Finally, if medical treatment fails surgery is sometimes helpful. The types of surgery available include synovectomy, reconstructive tendon surgery, arthroplasty and arthrodesis.
	Let me ask you one more question about treatment. What other line of treatment do you think Prince Charles would advise us to follow?
Student	You have floored me on this one. I really don't see what Prince Charles can have to do with the treatment of rheumatoid arthritis!
Consultant	Let me enlighten you. Prince Charles has a great interest in 'alternative' medicine, so what type of alternative approach is possible in RA?
Student	I'm still not sure.
Consultant	I'm referring to acupuncture which is claimed to relieve pain, stiffness and swelling of joints. Its place in the treatment of RA remains to be established by good clinical trials.
	To finish off Mrs S.'s treatment I want to ask you about her pyo-arthrosis.
Student	This should be treated by parenteral antibiotics according to the sensitivity of the organism found on culture.

OUTCOME

Pyo-arthrosis A penicillin-G sensitive *Staph. aureus* was isolated and Mrs S. was treated with 6-hourly intravenous penicillin for 4 weeks followed by oral amoxycillin 250 mg 8-hourly for a further month. The joint was also aspirated daily until no more fluid occurred. Joint pain was relieved rapidly, infection came under control within 48 hrs and there was full recovery in 6 weeks.

Rheumatoid arthritis Once the septic infection in the left knee was controlled it was possible to increase the dose of prednisolone very cautiously and with adequate physiotherapy the acute flare-up of the arthritis in the other joints progressively improved.

She was also given a blood transfusion of 2 units which increased her haemoglobin from 9.9 g/dl to 11.6 g/dl.

Subsequent progress Mrs S.'s progress over the next three years was satisfactory on a maintenance dose of 7.5 mg of enteric-coated prednisolone daily, and she was able to get back to limited housework.

She had two further acute flare-ups of the rheumatoid arthritis over this period, requiring a temporary increase in her daily dose of prednisolone to 30 mg, and settled satisfactorily on both occasions.

She adamantly refused to have any further injections of hydrocortisone into any of her joints!

LEARNING POINTS

Causes of polyarthritis

- rheumatoid arthritis
- osteo-arthritis
- gout
- psoriasis
- collagen disorders
     SLE
     systemic sclerosis
     polyarteritis nodosa
     mixed connective-tissue disease
- Reiter's disease
- gonorrhoea/chlamydia infection
- systemic disease
     inflammatory bowel disease
       ulcerative colitis
       Crohn's disease
     sarcoidosis
     amyloidosis
     malignancy

Pulmonary complications of RA

- pleurisy
- pleural effusion
- nodules of fibrosis (Caplan's syndrome — associated with pneumoconiosis)
- fibrosing alveolitis

Clinical features of SLE

- 'butterfly' rash
- lymphadenopathy and/or splenomegaly
- cardiac
     pericarditis
     endocarditis (Libman–Sacks disease)
- pleurisy with or without effusion
- peripheral neuritis
- glomerulonephritis

Auto-immune diseases which may be associated with RA

- inflammatory bowel disease
- diabetes
- pernicious anaemia
- Hashimoto's thyroiditis

Differentiation between RA and SLE

	RA	SLE
Patient	young/middle-aged woman	young woman
Onset	gradual	acute
Joints	small joints	small joints
	symmetrical	asymmetrical
Pain	constant	flitting
Morning stiffness	very common	absent
Deformity	common	rare
Systemic features	sometimes	frequent

Tests for RA

- blood count
    anaemia
        chronic infection
        gastrointestinal loss
        (a megaloblastic anaemia may also occur if the diet is inadequate)
    high WBC — watch out for sepsis
    high ESR
- X-ray joints
- serum for rheumatoid factor (positive in 80%)
- synovial fluid examination (especially if ? sepsis)

X-ray changes in the joints in RA

- juxta-articular osteoporosis
- narrow joint space due to loss of cartilage
- cystic erosions (may be marginal)
- dislocations and joint deformity

Synovial fluid analysis in RA and septic arthritis

	Rheumatoid arthritis	Septic arthritis
Appearance	cloudy yellow	cloudy green
Cells — WBC total	2000–75 000/mm^3	>100 000/mm^3
polymorphs	up to 50%	75% and over
Organisms	absent	present
Complement	low	normal

Treatment of RA

General
- bed rest
- treat anaemia (transfusion may be of temporary help if the anaemia is severe)

- immobilization of affected joints
- heat to relieve pain and stiffness
- wax baths for stiffness
- exercises to maintain muscle tone

Drugs
- first line
    - non-steroidal anti-inflammatory drugs
- second line
    - gold
    - penicillamine
    - antimalarials
        - chloroquine
        - hydroxychloroquine
    - sulphasalazine
- third line
    - steroids
- other
    - cytotoxic
        - azathioprine
        - cyclophosphamide

Side-effects of long-term steroids

- fluid retention
    - moon-face
    - ankle swelling
    - hypertension
    - heart failure (especially elderly)
- hypokalaemia (facilitates arrhythmias e.g. with digoxin)
- gastric irritation
    - indigestion
    - ulceration
    - blood loss
- diabetes
- osteoporosis with spontaneous fractures
- bruising
- psychosis
- Cushingoid features

Side-effects of gold and penicillamine

- rashes
- mouth ulcers
- gastro-enteritis
- nephrotic syndrome
- thrombocytopenia → pancytopenia

Indications for surgery in RA

- severe pain unresponsive to full medical treatment
- severe loss of essential joint function
- gross joint instability
- unacceptable loss of joint mobility
- progressive joint destruction on X-ray

Types of surgery available in RA

- synovectomy
- reconstructive tendon surgery
- arthroplasty
- arthrodesis

Index